For all the ex-cheerleaders toiling away in doctor's offices everywhere, without whom this book would not have been possible.

Introduction: The Woodcutter vs. The Perky Cheerleaders

I almost titled this book "The Pharmacy Bullshit List." Because That's what I think of the drugs I'm ready to write about. Bullshit.

But if I would have made that the first thing you see on the cover, a lot of you never would have picked up the book you're now holding, much less bought or borrowed or stole or whatever you did to get a copy, and I want to get this into the hands of as many people as possible. So, I softened the title a little. Of course, making "bullshit" the eighth word you see in the text probably isn't doing me any favors, but bullshit is what it is, and I'm tired of it. The frustration of watching rip offs disguised under a prescription label go out the pharmacy door for over 20 years has built up like lava under Krakatoa and I'm finally calling it. You can thank the woodcutter. Because it was the woodcutter and the look on his face on what would have been a normal workday that finally pushed me over the edge and eventually led to these words being in front of your eyes.

I should probably explain.

I'd pass by the woodcutter often on my way to the daily pharmacy grind. The city where I live and work has a place where they dump trees that get cut down in the course of city business. They drag them to a little pull off next to a secluded back road, then it's first come first serve free firewood. And there the woodcutter would be, almost as many days as not, working the pile with a simple hand axe. After awhile I noticed he was a regular customer in my pharmacy as well, and I chatted him up a little bit. I found out the guy worked construction and had been looking for work for the better part of a year now. This was during the depths of the recession of 2008, and I probably don't have to tell you that wasn't the best of times to be an unemployed construction worker. He said the wood dump was a godsend, as he couldn't afford his gas bill anymore and was dependent on his wood stove to heat his house. Then he handed me a prescription for Lotrel.

Lotrel is a medicine used to treat high blood pressure. Two medicines actually, both of which have been around awhile and are available as cheap as dirt generics. But since the woodcutter's prescription was made out for the combination product, we couldn't go the cheap as dirt route. The woodcutter's prescription was going to cost almost $80, and that was the generic version of the combination product. The brand name Lotrel cost almost two times that amount.

This was a man who just had his gas cut off. The look on the woodcutter's face said it all.

I asked him if he had a minute and picked up the phone. I waded through voicemail hell, sat on hold awhile, got cut off, started over and finally reached a nurse at his doctor's office. I asked her if we could just take this prescription and split it into one for each med. Sadly, I need a doctor's permission to do this even though the only difference is that the woodcutter would be taking two tablets instead of one.

The result? I got the woodcutter out the door for eighteen bucks. He wanted to hug me, but there is no hugging of this pharmacist. They used to call me the Drugnazi and there was a reason for that.

Unfortunately, the woodcutter's situation is hardly unique. While the pharmaceutical manufacturers never hesitate to tell you prescription prices are so high because of the staggering costs involved in discovering and bringing new medicines to market, the truth is, pharmacy shelves are also stocked with blatant rip offs. I'm not talking about different medicines in the same class with widely varying prices. The cholesterol lowering medication Crestor, for example, may cost a hundred dollars a month more than the generic version of its competitor Lipitor, but they are different medicines. While most people's cholesterol will be lowered just fine and their wallet left fatter with a Lipitor prescription, there are people out there who will respond better to Crestor.

I'm also not talking about the time-honored "extended

release" trick, where a drug company, just before a patent on one of its big sellers is about to expire, will introduce a new version of the same med that is taken less frequently and still priced at an arm and a leg. You can argue that there is some benefit to having to take your pills less often, and maybe it's worth it to some people to pay a price for that.

I'm not even talking about the "medical food" scheme. Let's say you want the prestige of a prescription drug without having to pay for all those time consuming and expensive tests the FDA requires to ensure it works and is safe. Or maybe you sell dietary supplements and feel constrained by regulations that say you cannot claim your product treats a specific disease. Is there a way you can overcome these hurdles you feel are holding you back from collecting more money?

Yes, you can call your product a food. Problem solved.

"Food?" you might be saying. "Like green beans? I don't see how green beans fit into this equation."

That's because you don't think like a business major.

The term "medical food" actually originated back in the 1950's, and referred to products such as baby formulas for patients with diseases that left them unable to process certain nutrients. Makes sense really. You come up with a product that meets the unique nutritional needs of people with certain diseases and they eat it. Like you or I would eat green beans. Around 2007 though, some clever marketers started to take advantage of the definition of "medical food." They would find a link to a disease and a type of vitamin, protein, or other food component. Any link. Not a proven link mind you, a good theory will do. They then put that vitamin or other food part in pill form and declare that the resulting product will only be sold with a doctor's recommendation. For example, there is a link between low levels of folate, a B vitamin, and depression. How significant this link is is a matter of debate among the medical community, and opinions vary. A company called Pamlab didn't wait for a consensus to develop or a theory to be proven though. They introduced a version of folate under the brand name Deplin. This product is sold in bottles that are full of tablets, not beans; it is marketed to health care professionals as a treatment to make antidepressants work better, and is sold only on a health professional's recommendation. So you go to the doctor because you're not feeling well, they give you a prescription they say will help, which you bring to me, and what you're buying is... legally food. Even though you could swallow a whole bottle and still be really hungry. Makes total sense, right?

And that Deplin will cost you over $3 a tablet. While traditional folate supplements, such as the folic acid you can find in any vitamin aisle, can be found in bottles of 250 for that same $3.

But even that doesn't rise to the level of total bullshit. Deplin is a slightly different form of folate than that folic acid, and you could make an argument that this different form will be of more benefit to a patient. A weak argument in my opinion, but one that some doctors who maybe went to Caribbean medical schools that had to be liberated by Reagan in the 80's, or perhaps are just easily influenced, might go for.

It takes a special kind of blatant rip off to make this pharmacist's bullshit list. Tiny manipulations of prescription strengths that make them no more effective but incredibly more expensive. Combination pills of meds that have been available separately for years treated as if they were a new product. A topical foam that contains the same product as a cream but is priced over a hundred dollars more. A glaucoma medicine that is repackaged with a little brush and sold, for more money, as an eyelash thickener. These are just some of the tricks used by the pharmaceutical industry to separate you from your money. There are others.

In fact, there has been a whole sub-industry develop in the last few years in the pharmaceutical world dedicated to milking money out of you and your insurance company by "researching" ways to repackage the familiar as the innovative. That is bullshit my friends, and when I saw the look on the woodcutter's face after I told him his prescription was $80, I couldn't take it anymore.

But here's the thing: I just don't have the time to contact your doctor to lobby for you the way I did for the woodcutter. I and almost everyone you see behind a pharmacy counter get stretched a little thinner every year, expected to squeeze out a few more prescriptions and jab a lot more flu shots with the same or fewer resources. And if I did have time to try to talk some sense into the prescribers of these highway robbery schemes disguised as medical advances, there's a chance they wouldn't want to hear it anyway.

Pharmaceutical companies are incredibly skilled at manipulating the people who prescribe their meds. Do you know the most common background of drug sales reps? Most of them aren't pharmacists, nurses, or doctors. Most aren't even people with a business background. The most common background for a pharmaceutical sales rep is college cheerleader. I am not making that up. There's a very good chance your doctor is learning everything they know about a new drug from a perky, bubbly, smoking hot ex-cheerleader who shows up at his office with a perky, bubbly, smoking hot smile, ready to lather attention and free food in exchange for a few minutes of face time. That's what we're up against, and I just can't save everyone who comes to my counter.

I can give you some information to arm yourself though. I've picked 50 of the most egregious, pointless, waste-of-money drugs you'll find in the pharmacy world and am giving you the lowdown in this book. If your doctor thinks any of them are right for you, you need to have a serious talk. There are exceptions to every rule, which means there might be instances where there is a good reason to prescribe one of these meds. They will be very rare. Don't leave your doctor's office unless and until you understand the reasoning behind their decision, and don't take the prescription unless and until you are convinced any advantage is worth the extra cash you or your insurance company will be paying for it. Remember, it's your body and your money.

And by the way, no matter how much money you might save by looking through these pages, don't hug me. Ever.

The prices I use here are always the result of a little shopping. I've looked over what a few of the major pharmacy chains and online drugstores are asking for the med, and I've done this for a reason. If you're lucky enough to have prescription coverage as part of your health insurance, the amount of money a pharmacy collects is determined by your insurance company, and will be the same no matter where the prescription is filled. For those of you on your own in paying your prescription bills however, prices from pharmacy to pharmacy can vary widely, so a little comparison shopping can save you a lot.

Here's something a little more surprising though - prices can also vary widely *within the same pharmacy*. Kind of like how every person on an airplane has paid a different price for their seat, it is possible for two people standing in line in a pharmacy at the same time, with the same prescription for the same medicine, to pay wildly different prices.

How? It all boils down to who has the right discount card.

Pay attention, because what I'm about to say may be the single most important tip in this book. Don't ever walk into a pharmacy without some sort of discount plan or card at your disposal. It'll take a little work and planning, but I promise you it will pay off. Many drug chains have in-house discount programs that will save you some dollars, but be careful. Features such as four dollar generics are great if you have a prescription on the four dollar list, but companies will make up those discounts somewhere, so watch out if you don't. Other chains charge money up front to be a member of their savings program, so you'll have to figure out if you'll still come out ahead. Other companies put out prescription discount cards at no charge that save you money off a pharmacy's full retail price. These cards sound too good to be true, but long story short, they allow a person to get the same discounts on prescriptions insurance companies negotiate for themselves. Both familywize.org and pharmacycard.org offer online price checkers that allow you to calculate what your prescription would cost using their discount cards. It'll take a little effort to determine whether a drugstore discount plan or an independent discount card is right for you, but it's worth it. I've seen customers save themselves $100 or more on a single prescription.

Back to my original point though, the prices I use here are meant to be used only as a tool to measure the bullshit. What you actually pay for a product could be more or less than the numbers I'm using. The point is to give you an idea of the scale of the financial shenanigans at play here, and to help cut through the bullshit, because I'm tired of it.

This is for the woodcutter.

Chapter 1: Acanya

The Med

Acanya is a topical gel used to treat acne that consists of two active ingredients: clindamycin, an antibiotic, and benzoyl peroxide, an agent that works as anti-bacterial by removing excess skin oil and dead skin cells that can clog pores.

Oh the horrors of teenage acne. The pock marked pizza face that strikes exactly when we are most insecure about our bodies and trying to socially establish ourselves. Only a stricken teenager, or possibly parent, can understand the anguish that goes through an adolescent's mind when confronted with zits in the mirror. I remember my teen years well, the creams and lotions, the scrubs and washes, the antibiotics and special diets. I went through it all, and I remember how I would have tried anything...*anything!!* to make my zits go away. Valeant Dermatology, the maker of Acanya, remembers as well, especially the part about being willing to do, or pay, anything.

The Scam

It's not that Acanya doesn't work, clindamycin and benzoyl peroxide are both recognized as effective in the treatment of acne, and both are cheap. A bottle of topical clindamycin goes for around 25 dollars. A tube of 10% benzoyl peroxide can be found over the counter in any drugstore's skin care section for around five.

Acanya, however, is anything but cheap. Packaged so it can pretend to be a new product, a tube of Acanya will set you back around $250. I'll leave it to you to decide if the convenience of only having to apply one cream instead of two is worth almost 10 times the price.

But wait, go to Acanya's web site and you'll see it touts big savings! Go there, and you can get a coupon so you'll pay only $25 if you have insurance. Your insurer gets stuck with the rest of the tab. Remember that the next time you're notified how much your rates are going up.

And if you're uninsured, or if your insurance company is smart enough not to fall for this, the "savings" plan will have you paying $50. The people at Valeant Dermatology are counting on you seeing that, after hearing the $250 regular price, and thinking you're getting quite the deal. I also imagine they're not too upset that a certain number of customers won't be savvy enough to hunt for special offers and therefore will end up paying full price.

Oh, one more thing. The benzoyl peroxide that's in Acanya is in a concentration of 2.5%, which is exactly 75% *weaker* than what you can buy on your own without a prescription. Acanya is a rip off.

What To Do

Don't fill a prescription for Acanya unless you have money burning a big hole in your pocket. Ask your doctor for a prescription for topical clindamycin instead, buy some benzoyl peroxide over the counter, and take the money you save and put it towards video games or cell phones or whatever the hell it is these kids are into nowadays.

Chapter 2: Altoprev

The Med

Altoprev is a brand of the popular cholesterol lowering medicine lovastatin, a generic drug sold for many years under the brand name Mevacor. Lovastatin was the first of the "statin" drugs to hit the market and was a huge advance in the treatment of heart disease. In 2009, over 200 million prescriptions were written for statins, and they have played a key role in the decline in the rate of cardiovascular related deaths over the last few decades.

The Scam

Altoprev is different from the other forms of lovastatin on the market in that it is an extended-release form of the drug. This may confuse some of you who just read the introduction to this book, as I just said the "extended release" trick is a fairly common one drug companies use to get some extra years out of a patent monopoly, and those drugs wouldn't make the cut. One could make an argument that taking a med less often could have a therapeutic benefit. It's easier to remember to take a pill once a day than twice a day or more after all. In this case though, Altoprev is an extended-release version of a medicine that is usually prescribed to be taken... once a day. I'll say that again to let that sink in. Altoprev is an extended release product that is made in the same strength, and taken just as often as the immediate release version it competes with.

In its official prescribing information, the maker of Altoprev, Shionogi Inc., goes to great lengths to show that the absorption of once a day Altoprev is smoother and steadier than absorption of a once a day regular lovastatin tablet. But does that matter? After all, you take a statin to lower your cholesterol, not to produce elegant looking graphs of drug levels. So, is there a cholesterol lowering advantage to Altoprev?

In that same package insert, Shionogi implies there is. It shows a chart that tells a tale of increased cholesterol lowering effectiveness. A 29.6% reduction in "bad" cholesterol (LDL) versus a 24% reduction using an equal dose of regular lovastatin for instance. Except, the data for Altoprev comes from a grand total of 34 people, while the lovastatin study cited used over 1600, making any comparison between the two an exercise in statistical garbage. Even if this weren't the case however, you would pay dearly for that rather small difference. A month of the most common strength of Altoprev will most likely cost you over $350. A month of the immediate release lovastatin can easily be had for less than ten. That's a lot of money to spend for a product whose numbers have to be massaged almost to the point of breaking even to claim the smallest of benefits.

What To Do

If your doctor writes you a prescription for Altoprev, politely ask for the immediate release lovastatin instead. Even if it turns out lovastatin doesn't get your cholesterol to where it needs to be, the answer almost certainly won't be using an extended release form instead. There are more powerful and still inexpensive relatives of lovastatin that would have a much bigger impact on your clinical outcome than Altapro ever would. Stay away from Altoprev and your heart will be happy. Not because of your cholesterol level, but because your wallet will be full.

Chapter 3: Androgel 1.62%

The Med

Androgel is a topical form of testosterone, and testosterone, in the eyes of the drug marketers, is the new estrogen. When I first became a pharmacist the estrogen flowed through our store like water in the mighty Mississippi. Premarin, Estrace, Cenestin, and all their friends were touted as a way to counter the symptoms of menopause; the hot flashes, mood swings, and insomnia that often come with the end of menstrual cycles. The bestselling book "Feminine Forever" went even further. Its author, Dr. Robert A. Wilson, wrote in 1966 that with estrogen therapy, a woman's:

> *"breasts and genital organs will not shrivel. She will be much more pleasant to live with and will not become dull and unattractive."*

Well who wouldn't want a piece of that? No wonder that river of estrogen was flowing out the door.

But then it was demonstrated there was a link between estrogen therapy and breast cancer. Sales shriveled like the ovaries of the good Dr. Wilson's imagination, and the fact estrogen was no longer being passed out like candy is credited with a 10% drop in the rate of breast cancer from 2000 to 2004. What's a drug industry to do when a cash cow is linked to a potentially life threatening illness?

Work on the other sex.

I can hardly remember seeing a male customer on any hormone therapy when I first started my time behind the pharmacy counter, but these days it seems as if a testosterone river has replaced the estrogen flows of old. The numbers back up what I see, with sales of testosterone products up more than 500% since 1993, according to medicinenet.com. Drugs like Androgel are touted as ways to build muscle, sharpen memory and concentration, boost sex drive, and improve energy levels.

Well who wouldn't want a piece of that? Wait. I think I remember seeing a show like this before. And I don't like how that one ended.

As long as this show goes on though, Androgel plans on being a part of it.

The Scam

The makers of Androgel, Abbott Labs, recently introduced a concentrated version of the product. There are now two strengths on the market, 1% and 1.62%. The average starting dose of the concentrated version is two pumps a day, as opposed to four for the older 1% strength. Abbott also cut the price by around $17 a month.

"That's not much of a scam," you may be saying, and you would be right, for now. This is more of a slow motion scam whose trap is yet to be sprung. The older 1% concentration is set to lose its patent protection in 2016 you see, so by luring as many people as possible to the new strength that no one claims is any more effective, Abbott is hoping by the time a generic 1% competitor comes to the market, there will be no customers left to use it. By offering you that $17 discount now, it plans to keep you or your insurance company paying over $300 a month for your increased libido long past the point when you could be getting the same results for less.

What To Do

Happily take Abbott up on its cheaper 1.62% strength for now. Seventeen dollars a month is $204 a year after all. But when the generic competitors to the 1% show up, ask your doctor to switch to the 1%. And don't take no for an answer. Unless you're the type of person who puts a lot of value on pumping two fewer times a day.

Chapter 4:
Antara/Fenoglide

The Meds

Antara and Fenoglide are both forms of the anti-cholesterol drug fenofibrate. Two of many fenofibrate forms, as we'll see very soon. The benefits of keeping cholesterol at a normal level in the prevention of heart attacks, strokes, and other cardiovascular diseases is well documented, and fenofibrate plays an important part in the war on cholesterol, with millions of prescriptions written per year. Finding a fenofibrate that won't break the bank or your heart is the challenge though, as you're about to see.

The Scam

Trying to keep up with the fenofibrate market isn't easy. It all started simply enough in 1998, when Abbott labs introduced the med under the brand name Tricor in three different strengths: 67, 134, and 200 milligrams. Sadly for Abbott, by the time Tricor made it to market, its patent was set to run out only two years later. What's a drug company to do when it only has a couple years to enjoy monopoly pricing on one of its products? Shrug its shoulders and say "Oh well, that's the way capitalism works sometimes," and get to work researching and developing the next breakthrough cholesterol medicine? If that's what you're thinking, you're obviously not a capitalist or research scientist working for the pharmaceutical industry. Because the way Abbott handled its little Tricor problem is a lesson in the innovative ways of the American free market.

First, it sued the company planning to bring a generic version of Tricor to market. This would allow them to keep things tied up in the courts for a couple of years at least.

Then, they simply stopped making the old strengths of Tricor, and replaced them with 54 and 160mg versions. They then deployed their army of sales reps to medical offices around the country to pretend like these new strengths of Tricor were a brand new product. We'll call it Tricor the second.

Within six months 97 percent of fenofibrate prescriptions were for the new Tricor, which was not substitutable for the original. By the time the generic drug makers were able to get their version of the original Tricor to market, it was too late. No one was writing for it.

Was this because Tricor the second was better? Nope. Abbott didn't submit a single study to show that its new Tricor worked any better than its old Tricor. Was it because Tricor the second was a better value? If you think that I haven't taught you a single thing by writing this book. Remember how I told you earlier that the single most common background for drug industry sales reps was college cheerleader? I'm guessing the popularity of the new Tricor might have had something to do with perky personalities and cleavage.

Eventually though, generic drug manufacturers petitioned the FDA to let them make Tricor the second, and Abbott again sued to keep things tied up in court a couple years. Any guesses on what they did next? Out came Tricor the third, now in 48 and 145mg versions, without a lick of proof that they work any better than Tricor the first or second.

Seventy days after the introduction of Tricor the third it accounted for 70 percent of fenofibrate prescriptions. By the time the generic companies caught up with Tricor the second, Tricor the third had 96 percent of the market.

Since there was no longer a patent on fenofibrate itself, other drug companies eventually decided that they wanted to get in on this "slightly different version of Tricor" action, with the result being that at the time of this writing, fenofibrate is now available in 40, 43, 45, 48, 50, 54, 67, 120, 130, 134, 160, and 200 milligram versions. Keep in mind no medical person ever said there was a need for any other strengths of fenofibrate back when the original Tricor came in only three. This explosion of fenofibrate was driven by financial factors only. Say what you will about the pharmaceutical industry, but it truly innovates like no other.

So where do Antara and Fenoglide fit into all of this? They are currently the only versions of fenofibrate that the generic makers haven't caught up to. You'll pay about $80 a month for the lower strengths of these products, 40 and 43 milligrams, respectively, while a generic version of Tricor the second (54mg) will run you or your insurance company around $25. That's over three times as much a month, for less drug. The higher strengths will lighten your wallet even more, costing you or your insurance company around $180 a month more than you could be paying. Antara and Fenoglide didn't start the fenofibrate rip-off game, but they are currently the biggest winners.

What To Do

If you get a prescription for Tricor or any of the other forms of fenofibrate, it'll pay to do your homework. Currently the best deals are on Tricor the second, (54 and 160 milligrams) which will cost you or your insurance from around 25 to 50 dollars a month, depending on which strength your prescriber decides you need. Compare that with the $230 thirty days of Fenoglide can cost you and you could find yourself heartbroken, no matter what your cholesterol level.

Chapter 5: Aplenzin

The Med

Aplenzin is a brand name of the drug bupropion, which has been a mainstay in the treatment of depression for over 20 years. It works differently from the popular meds such as Prozac, Zoloft, Celexa, and Paxil, known as SSRI inhibitors, which has allowed it to develop a niche as an alternative or add on medicine when a patient's response to an SSRI is not adequate or side effects are a problem. Bupropion was also approved for use as a smoking cessation aid after studies showed it almost doubled the chances a person would successfully quit smoking. The vast majority of bupropion prescriptions are written to treat depression though, and with an estimated 17% of the American population battling depression at some point in their lives, it's a huge, multi-billion dollar market.

The Scam

While bupropion has been on the market for almost a generation, Aplenzin has not. It was introduced by Sanofi-Aventis in 2009 as bupropion *hydrobromide,* slightly different than the bupropion *hydrochloride* that has been sold under the brand name Wellbutrin since the 80's. This slight difference is enough to keep any prescription written for Aplenzin from being filled with a generic version of Wellbutrin, but not enough to keep it from working any differently. Both brands of bupropion are bioequivalent, which means they put the same amount of medicine into your bloodstream at the same rate. In fact, Sanofi-Aventis doesn't make any claims that Aplenzin works any better or is any safer than other forms of bupropion, the only advantage they tout in their promotional literature is that since Wellbutrin doesn't come in a strength equal to the maximum daily dose of bupropion and Aplenzin does, if you need that maximum dose you can take one tablet instead of two. That's it. Aplenzin is no more effective than any other form of bupropion. It is no safer. It's just if you need a high dose, you can take one tablet instead of two.

How much do you pay for that privilege? A month of the highest strength of Aplenzin costs almost $600. And even though you would have to get two prescriptions for two different strengths of Wellbutrin to get the maximum daily dose, you would pay around $90 for the generic version of both.

But why does it look like you're getting more medicine with Aplenzin versus Wellbutrin? After all, the label on the highest dose of Aplenzin says 522 milligrams, while the maximum dose of Wellbutrin is 450 milligrams. Surely 522 is more than 450, right?

The people at Sanofi-Aventis might not mind if you thought so, but the answer is no. Remember the only difference between Aplenzin and Wellbutrin is the ion the bupropion is attached to, bupropion *bromide* instead of bupropion *chloride*. Since bromine weighs more than chlorine, coupling bupropion with a bromide ion results in a molecule that weighs more, even though it contains the same amount of bupropion. Don't be fooled by the numbers. You're getting the same amount of medicine either way.

What to do

Spending over $6000 a year that I didn't have to would be enough to make me depressed over the condition of my wallet. If you feel the same way, and you don't mind taking more than one tablet at a time, kindly ask your doctor to change a prescription for Aplenzin to one for Wellbutrin. Chances are your outlook on life will start to improve once you see your total at the pharmacy counter.

Chapter 6: Aricept 23

The Med

Aricept, the brand name of donepezil, is a member of a class of meds known as cholinesterase inhibitors. It works by increasing the amount of acetylcholine in the brain, and has become a cornerstone of Alzheimer's therapy. While not a cure, it can delay the progression of symptoms and is one of the limited options available to sufferers of the disease. As such it became a blockbuster seller for its makers, the Japanese company Eisai and their American partners Pfizer, generating over $2 billion in annual revenue. It was set to lose its patent protection in November of 2010 however, which would lead the way for generic competition.

The Scam

I almost didn't list the meds in this book alphabetically, because I wanted to save this one for last, as it crosses a line I thought would never be crossed. Aricept was available for years in 5 and 10 milligram strengths. Shortly before its patent protection was set to expire however, Eisai and Pfizer applied for approval of a 23 milligram version.

"What an odd number" you may be saying to yourself. Notice how that odd number cannot be reached by using the soon to be cheap 5 and 10 mg strengths.

Still, it is intuitive that a higher dose of medication would improve clinical outcomes. Science doesn't run on intuition though, in science things have to be proven, so a study was started. The FDA set a benchmark that said the new strength had to improve both cognitive (mental) and global (overall) function in Alzheimer's patients in order to be approved.

Aricept 23 flunked. The study showed only slight improvement in cognitive function and no improvement at all in global function. The FDA however, against the advice of both a clinical and statistical reviewer, approved Aricept 23 anyway. The New York Times reported that Dr. Russell Katz, director of the F.D.A.'s neurology products division, "acknowledged side effects from the higher dose 'could lead to significant morbidities and even increased mortality,' but concluded that the drug most likely improved overall functioning even though the study did not show that."

Two points about what just happened here:

1) "but concluded that the drug most likely improved overall functioning even though the study did not show that." So much for science not running on intuition, as the intuition of the right person was what got this drug approved. The medical professions have become used to numbers being massaged, facts being twisted, and any and everything possible being done to put a med in the best light possible in the scientific literature, but this

is the first time I'm aware of when they've given up on even pretending like the scientific facts matter. "The study did not show that," and it still didn't matter.

2) Which might be forgivable if it were done in the name of trying anything possible to help the victims of a terrible disease. But Katz also "acknowledged side effects could lead to significant morbidities and even increased mortality." Just to be clear, morbidity is a fancy word for sickness. Mortality is one for death.

So the FDA approved a drug that did not meet its criteria for effectiveness, and that its head of neurology products said may leave more people dead. That's the story of Aricept 23 in one sentence.

Oh, and Aricept 23 costs about 90 dollars a month more than the safer and effective 10mg generic version.

What To Do

Let me be clear: Aricept 5 and 10mg are perfectly appropriate choices for Alzheimer's patients. It's only when the dose went up to 23mg that it crossed the line into bullshit. There may be isolated cases where a dose that high is beneficial, but they tried to prove its effectiveness at that dose and got marginal results. What Aricept 23 does do is more than triple the incidence of nausea and vomiting, increase by 60 percent the chance of diarrhea, and depletes your loved one's assets by over a thousand dollars a year. Unless there is a good reason not to, stick with the lower doses.

Chapter 7: Atralin

The Med

Atralin is a brand name for the topical acne medicine tretinoin, and tretinoin was my teenage savior. Regular use, a little peeling to let me know I was using too much, a sunburn or two to teach me those warning stickers put on by the pharmacy weren't just for show, and the volcanic mountain range that had erupted on my face eventually went into submission. The fact tretinoin can make acne worse before it makes it better was a little disconcerting, but after a few weeks, this pimply faced future professional was convinced tretinoin was a gift from heaven. I was now free to become socially awkward based only on the merits of my actions and not on the condition of my skin. It felt better somehow to know my awkwardness was now earned.

To make it even better, as I approach middle age, tretinoin has now also come into wide use in the treatment of facial wrinkles, making it easy to think of it as some sort of lifetime sex appeal in a tube. There are some people who would pay a lot for lifetime sex appeal, no questions asked I bet. Valeant Dermatology, the same company that brought us the rip-off acne med Acanya I talked about earlier, seems to have made that bet as well.

The Scam

Some of you more astute readers may have read the above description of tretinoin and wondered if I wasn't talking about Retin-A. I was. Retin-A was the original topical tretinoin, and is now saving the complexions of the children of its first generation of users. Drugs this old have generally lost their patent protection and are available as money-saving generics, and Retin-A is no exception. Funny thing about this med though, even though it's sold in different strengths, including 0.05%, and even though it's available in both a cream and a gel formulation, one way you can't get it is as a 0.05% gel. This is where Valeant saw its opportunity. It introduced Atralin, a 0.05% gel form of tretinoin and marketed it as a new product not substitutable for a generic. The price? $250 for a 45 gram tube. Over four times the price I found for the same size 0.05% cream with a little shopping around.

Neither the cream nor the gel has been shown to be more effective by the way. Keep that in mind when you're making your purchasing decisions.

Once again however, a little looking around will lead you to a "savings offer," where insured patients, most insured patients that is, will pay $25. If you're one of the lucky ones who qualifies for that $25 copay though, just remember your pharmacy has submitted a claim to your insurer for $250. Uninsured patients will pay $75 with the savings card. Which means Atralin is a product whose primary purpose it would seem, is to drain money away from your insurance company and those people not savvy enough to look for coupons, and into the coffers of Valeant Dermatology.

What To Do

Unless you're just a really big fan of topical gels, there's little if any reason to buy Atralin. Just stick with the generic Retin-A.

Actually, let me take that back. The box design on the generic tretinoins can be a bit boring. They have plain old boxy letters and tired plain color schemes. So if it's important to you to have stylish graphic artwork in your medicine cabinet, then by all means, go for the Atralin.

The rest of us though, can take the money we save on our lifetime sex appeal in a tube and spend it wining and dining our soon to be many suitors.

Chapter 8: Bidil

The Med

Bidil is a combination of two medications, hydralazine and isosorbide, used to treat heart failure, defined as when the heart cannot pump enough blood to meet the needs of the body. It works by dilating blood vessels, thereby lessening the amount of work required to move blood through the cardiovascular system. Heart failure is a horrible condition to have and an awful way to die. The memory of an afflicted patient I was assigned to study in college lying in his hospital bed day after day gasping for breath was all it took for me to make sure I started taking my blood pressure medicine regularly when I was diagnosed ten years later. If you have hypertension, which is one of the leading causes of heart failure, you should too, as the prognosis for heart failure patients is not good. While there are treatments that can improve a patient's symptoms and quality of life, the only cure is to undergo a heart transplant. Bidil however, has a unique role in the treatment of this condition. It was the first prescription product approved for a specific race, gaining approval from the FDA in 2005 for use specifically in African Americans after a study showed the drug combo to be more effective for black patients and that other heart failure drugs might not be as effective in African Americans as they are in whites.

The Scam

At first, this would seem to be the type of thing health care research should be all about. Practical news we can use to deliver the optimal outcome for each individual patient. The problem comes when it's time to pay the bill. Both hydralazine and isosorbide have been around for a long time, and are cheap as dirt. You'll pay just four dollars a month for a supply of each at one of the country's major drug retailers. Present them with a prescription for Bidil though, and it's possible you'll be expected to fork over close to $70.

Is Bidil more expensive to make than regular hydralazine and isosorbide? No. It's the exact same thing, with one little twist. Bidil uses a strength of hydralazine, 37.5 milligrams, not otherwise available commercially. This means the generic can't be used without a specific authorization from your doctor.

One again however, the manufacturer of an overpriced, unsubstitutable medication, in this case Arbor Pharmaceuticals, is offering a "savings program" to people willing to make an effort to look for bargains. Some people will make out OK for themselves with this deal, as people whose insurance will cover Bidil will end up with a $0 copay. Great for you, bad for your insurance company which just got stuck with a $840 annual drug bill. Probably also bad for your future health insurance premiums, as insurance companies tend to get back the dollars they pay out, and then some.

Uninsured patients pay $25 a month under Arbor's "savings program," which sounds like a great deal compared to the regular retail price, but is still almost three times as much as buying both medicines separately at a pharmacy with a four dollar generic program. That's almost $200 extra a year you'll be paying for nothing other than taking one tablet at a time as opposed to two.

What To Do

While there is not a 37.5 milligram strength of hydralazine on the market, it is available in 25 and 50 milligram versions. Ask your doctor if she thinks either one is appropriate for you, and if so, have her write out two separate prescriptions for isosorbide and hydralazine and start thinking what you'll do with the money you've saved.

Chapter 9: Binosto

The Med

Binosto is an effervescent version of the drug alendronate, used to treat the bone thinning disease osteoporosis. The exact role of this class of meds, known as bisphosphonates, and how they should be used is subject to some controversy, and it's not my intention to go into the specifics here. What isn't in doubt though, is that alendronate and the other bisphosphonates have an important role to play in the treatment of what can be a devastating disease.

The Scam

Alendronate has been around for years, gaining popularity under the brand name Fosamax and available in a generic version since 2008. The Binosto difference is that effervescence, which means you drop it into a glass of water and it fizzes while it dissolves, just like the Alka Seltzer we all know and love. Is Binosto an improvement over the older versions of alendronate? I guess that would depend on your definition of "improvement."

You have to be careful to protect your esophagus while taking the older versions of alendronate, making sure you stand or sit upright for at least 30 minutes after taking a dose. The same thing applies to Binosto.

While bisphosphonates strengthen the bones of the hip and spine, there have also been reports linking them to the death of bone in the jaw, as well as fractures of the femur. All the same precautions and warnings about this that apply to regular alendronate apply to Binosto as well.

So what exactly does Binosto add to bisphosphonate treatment options? It's fizzy. You put it in a glass of water and watch it fizz. That's it. I suppose there are some people out there who might find fizzy tablets entertaining, and I won't judge them for that. I will let you know however, that a month's supply of Binosto will cost around $150, while you should be able to find a month's worth of generic alendronate for somewhere between 10 to 15 dollars.

Actually there is another Binosto difference. An effervescent tablet is loaded with sodium, which I guess would make Binosto a great choice for someone on a high sodium diet. *(Note: I have never seen anyone put on a high sodium diet.)*

What To Do

The choice here is simple. If your doctor wants to prescribe Binosto, ask about a prescription for generic alendronate instead. Binosto is no safer. It is no more or less effective. It's just fizzy.

If you're watching your salt intake as part of a plan to keep your blood pressure under control, than all that sodium does make a difference, as one Binosto tablet alone contains almost 30% of the daily recommended sodium intake. The choice here is simple as well. Stay away from Binosto, period.

If you're the type of person who's willing to pay top dollar for fizzy based entertainment though, your choices might be a little more complicated. You could spend an extra $1620 a year on Binosto, but you might think about just picking up some Alka-Seltzer. You'd get all the fizz for a fraction of the price.

The choice is yours.

Chapter 10: Caduet

The Med

Heart disease and strokes are the number one and four killers of Americans, taking over 700,000 lives in 2009 according to the Center for Disease control and prevention. Fearsome as they are, medical science has made great progress in treating both conditions.

Advances in dietary recommendations, documenting the importance of exercise in keeping both hypertension (high blood pressure) and cholesterol under control, and the introduction of new medications all contributed to an almost 30% decline in cardiovascular related deaths from 1999 to 2009. And when I say new medications, I mean lots of medications. I could name a dozen drugs to control high blood pressure off the top of my head, and with a little thought, I'm sure I could come up with a dozen cholesterol drugs as well. Caduet combines one of each in the same tablet, the antihypertensive med amlodipine, sold for years under the brand name Norvasc, and the cholesterol lowering drug atorvastatin, sold under the name Lipitor. Both were blockbusters in their respective categories, generating over 15 billion dollars in sales for their manufacturer, Pfizer, while saving a lot of lives. It was a win-win situation, until the patents for Norvasc and Lipitor ran out that is, when generic competition would start to eat into the river of dollars flowing Pfizer's way.

The Scam

So what's a drug company to do when it's looking at the end of that type of revenue stream? Crank up the research machine, that's what. Not research into finding new and improved meds to take the place of Norvasc and Lipitor mind you, more like looking into ways to convince doctors that writing a prescription for one tablet that combined the two meds was better than writing two prescriptions for each individual drug. There might be some value in taking fewer tablets at a time, but at around $190 dollars a month for the most common strength, Caduet is priced $170 more than you would pay for individual prescriptions of amlodipine and atorvastatin. That's $2040 a year for the privilege of taking one tablet at a time instead of two.

Once again though, there is a drug manufacturer "savings card" that claims to soften the blow. This one though, mostly serves to just pour salt in your wounded wallet. Pfizer calls it the "Caduet $4 copay card" which may lead you to believe you'll be paying only four dollars for your prescription. You probably won't. Reading the fine print of their offer you'll see this:

> "By using the Card, patients will pay a minimum of $4 per refill and receive savings of up to $125 per refill."

What does that mean? It means if you have good insurance, you might end up paying $4 and sticking your insurer for the rest. For everyone else though, the "$4 copay card" just takes $125 off your bill. Remember, the most common strength of Caduet costs around $190. So when you come to the pharmacy with a "$4 copay card," you will leave after paying $65. And if you're unlucky enough to need the highest strength, that "$4 copay card" can lead to a pharmacy bill of $140. Pfizer's research department has evidently been hard at work, discovering some sort of new math.

What To Do

"Caduet is not for everyone" says its official website "It is not for those with liver problems. And it is not for women who are nursing, pregnant, or may become pregnant." I would add that it is also not for anyone who values money even a little bit. I can't think of a single reason to justify the existence of Caduet other than corporate greed. If your doctor tries to give you a prescription for this revenue enhancer in pill form, tell him you'll take it if he'll pay you the difference between that promised $4 copay and what you'll actually have to cough up to get the prescription filled. Otherwise have him write you out a prescription for amlodipine and one for atorvastatin.

Unless for some reason you really, really want to just take one pill instead of two.

Chapter 11: Clarinex

The Med

Clarinex is the brand name for the allergy medicine desloratadine. It belongs to the class known as antihistamines, and for those of you who don't know, histamine is the compound in your body responsible for the itchy eyes, the runny nose, the sneezing, and the general yuckiness that comes from an allergic reaction. As the name implies, an antihistamine works against the effects of histamine, which can seem like a gift from heaven above when allergies strike. Antihistamines are among the largest selling category of drugs ever, with several prescription and over the counter options available to help allergy sufferers cope. The early antihistamines all had a problem though. They made people drowsy. A lot of people. So many as a matter of fact that someone got the idea to slap another label on them and market them as sleep aids. Check the label of most any over the counter sleep aid and Benadryl Allergy and you will see they contain the exact same ingredient. This problem was solved in 1993 with the approval of loratadine, sold under the brand name Claritin. Loratadine is a non-sedating antihistamine that became the mother of all blockbuster drugs for Schering-Plough, now part of drug giant Merck.

The Scam

Some of you probably noticed how similar the words desloratadine and loratadine are to each other. There's a reason for that. Loratadine you see, is changed into desloratadine in the body as part of the normal metabolism process, and it's the desloratadine that actually blocks the effects of histamine. In other words, loratadine doesn't start to work until it is changed by your liver into desloratadine, its active metabolite.

So why not just cut out the middleman, right? That's the idea behind Clarinex. Except, that idea didn't seem to come to the people of Schering-Plough until that blockbuster Claritin of theirs had changed from a $100 a month prescription product into an over-the-counter med available anywhere drugs are sold for less than $10. Only when that revenue river became a tiny little dribble did the smart minds at Schering-Plough realize maybe that middleman could be cut, that a new patent could be applied for and desloratadine could be marketed as a new drug that might recapture some of that Claritin revenue stream. Only then was Clarinex born.

The price? Over $150 a month. Or you can go generic and knock that down to maybe $50, which sounds like a great deal until you remember that regular loratadine, which as you'll recall is converted into desloratadine, can be had over the counter for around $10.

What To Do

The great thing about this scam is that if your doctor does hand you a prescription for Clarinex, you won't need them to do a thing to avoid it. You won't even need your pharmacist to get involved. Simply head to the drugstore and go to the allergy aisle. Pick up some Claritin, or ideally the store's house brand, and save yourself over $100.

"But if I do that and the Claritin doesn't seem to work, then I should have that Clarinex prescription filled, right?" some of you may be saying. The answer would be no. Clarinex is simply the result of Claritin going through your liver remember, so if one doesn't work the chances that the other will are essentially zero. You'll see when you're in that allergy aisle saving yourself from a huge prescription bill, that there are several over the counter allergy treatments these days. Zyrtec and Allegra took a cue from Claritin's jump to over the counter status and now compete with them for shelf space. Different people respond to different meds, so if Claritin isn't cutting it for you, try one of the others until you find one that does the job. Other options include products such as Tavist or Chlor-Trimeton, but with these you'll run the risk of drowsiness.

And if you're looking for allergy relief as well as a sleep aid? Then Benadryl will be like two drugs in one.

Clarinex though, is best left behind the pharmacy counter to collect dust, and dust is one of the major triggers of allergies. Which is a little ironic when you think about it.

Chapter 12: Colcrys

The Med

Colcrys is the brand name for colchicine, a mainstay in the treatment of gout, and many of you who have had colchicine prescriptions over the years may be surprised to see it listed here. You may remember the med as a cheap, effective remedy for the searing pain that was in your big toe, and for many years you were right. Too many years. That's part of the story. To say colchicine is as old as time itself would only be a slight exaggeration, as references to the use of colchicine containing plants in medicine go all the way back to ancient Egypt. That's the problem. When an ancient medicine meets a modern government bureaucracy, guess who wins? Hint: not you.

The Scam

For many years in this country marketing medicine was a wild west-like affair. It wasn't until 1906 that there was any legal requirement that medicines not be adulterated or misbranded. It wasn't until 1938 that drugs were required to be proven safe, and not until 1962 that there was any requirement that they be shown to be effective. In both 1938 and 1962 however, drugs that were already on the market were "grandfathered in," or allowed to continue to be sold without going through the new regulatory hoops. That started to change in 2006, when the FDA started an initiative to hold all drugs to post-1962 standards.

What did that mean? It meant that to continue to be sold, every med that had been grandfathered in now had to go through the new drug approval process, going through the same hoops that a drug discovered this week has to go through.

Drugs discovered this week though, are way more expensive than drugs that have been around since the time of the pyramids. This wasn't a consideration of the FDA when they started this initiative.

So, for the price of a few studies that showed colchicine to be more effective than a placebo, that there was a better way to dose it than the way it was usually done, and pointed out a couple drug interactions, URL Pharma was granted a patent that treated colchicine as a brand new medicine. They started to sell it under the brand name Colcrys, and what was once cheap as dirt now sells for over five dollars a tablet, as all older, unapproved versions of colchicine have been removed from the market. Your tax burden may have been reduced over the last three decades, as the income tax cuts that started with the Reagan administration have reduced the top marginal rate from 70 to 39.6 percent, but your government is still effective in coming up with ways to separate you from your money. Same med, same strength, and thanks to the FDA and URL Pharma, now over 50 times more expensive.

What To Do

Unfortunately URL Pharma has a corner on the colchicine market until its patent expires in 2028, which means if you need it, you're stuck. There's a chance you may not need it though. If you're taking Colcrys regularly to prevent gout, ask your doctor if they think you would be helped by another drug, allopurinol, which has been around for years and sells for about $150 a month less. If you definitely need colchicine though, the best you can do is to head to Colcrys' web site, where you can find coupons that will keep you (but not your insurance company) from paying full retail price.

Chapter 13: Dolgic Plus

The Med

If reading my writing to this point has done nothing but give you a giant headache, than Dolgic Plus may be the med for you. It's actually not one med, but three. First is butalbital, a barbiturate being used here to relax the muscle contractions involved in a tension headache. Second is the popular over the counter pain reliever acetaminophen, which you're probably familiar with by the brand name Tylenol. Last is caffeine. Yes, caffeine. It's being used here not to give you your morning kick, but because there is evidence that a dose of caffeine can add to the effects of painkillers to get rid of a headache. The combination has been used in some form to combat headaches since long before I ever set foot behind a pharmacy counter.

The Scam

Not, however in the particular form found in Dolgic Plus. The most common strength of butalbital/acetaminophen/caffeine combination is a 50/325/40 milligram tablet. A version with 500mg acetaminophen is also available. Dolgic pushes the acetaminophen envelope a little further however, giving you 750mg per tablet.

That's it. The difference between Dolgic and its most

popular competitor is less than the amount of acetaminophen in a tablet of Extra Strength Tylenol.

How much will you pay for the Dolgic difference? Thirty tablets will most likely set you back over $150, while the same number of the 50/325/40mg tablets would be around $15.

Which means my writing really must be giving you a headache if you think Dolgic Plus is worth it.

What To Do

Try to keep focused and think clearly, even though you're in pain, and when you see the word "Dolgic" on a prescription paper, ask the prescriber to change it to Fioricet instead. It'll be substituted at the pharmacy for the 50/325/40mg generic, and you'll have more than a hundred extra dollars in your pocket. If you really want that extra acetaminophen, buy yourself some over the counter regular strength Tylenol, take a tablet with each Fioricet dose, and you'll still have more than a hundred extra dollars in your pocket. And a pain free head.

Maybe then you'll even decide to make it the rest of the way through this book.

Chapter 14: Doryx

The Med

Doryx is an enteric coated version of the antibiotic doxycycline, which has been around since the 1960's and is used to treat a wide variety of infections, from sinusitis to rectal Chlamydia and many things in between, including infections of the respiratory tract and skin, syphilis, Legionnaires disease, anthrax, and Lyme disease. Doxycycline could have stopped the Black Death of Europe's Middle Ages and is useful in the prevention of malaria. Doryx, though, is marketed exclusively for the treatment of acne, possibly the most common indication for doxycycline. Doryx is the same drug doctors and pimple plagued teenagers have known and used for years, with one twist, the enteric coating. This type of coating on a tablet keeps it from starting to dissolve until it has passed through your stomach and has entered your intestines, the idea being that this will reduce stomach upset. It's a theory that makes sense, but one that hasn't actually been proven in Doryx's case.

The Scam

Still, if doxycycline is upsetting your stomach, an enteric coated product like Doryx might be worth a try, right? In theory, yes.

The problem is the price. One month of Doryx will cost you or your insurance company somewhere in the neighborhood of $500. You read that correctly - over $6000 a year to treat your complexion.

And don't think they're asking you to pay this kind of money because making enteric coated tablets is an expensive thing to do. You can buy a bottle of 120 enteric coated aspirin tablets for less than $6.

One bit of good news is that Doryx has been around long enough now that it is available as a money saving generic. Good news is relative of course, and while that generic does lower the price by around 20%, that still would leave you paying somewhere in the neighborhood of $400 a month. Another is that Doryx's manufacturer, Warner Chilcott, offers a "savings card" that claims to lower your out of pocket expense to $25 and sock your insurance company with the rest. However, the fine print in the "savings card" offer does say "Maximum reimbursement levels apply," which is telling you there are people in the program who may end up paying more than that advertised $25, so buyer beware. I'll also point out again that insurance companies usually do have ways of getting back the dollars you sock them with.

Also, lest you think that doxycycline is just an expensive medication, I'll tell you a month of the regular doxycycline that we've all known and loved for almost 40 years will cost you around $12.

You read that correctly. Warner Chilcott took a cheap as dirt drug, added a coating to the tablets, and marked up the price over 4000%.

What To Do

Unless you have taken doxycycline and found it to be too hard on your stomach, there is no reason to take Doryx. It is no more effective, side effects are identical, and the end results will be the same. That enteric coating is the only difference. Which means unless you know or have reason to believe that regular doxycycline will be hard on your stomach, if your doctor hands you a prescription for Doryx, you should hand it right back.

If doxycycline does make your tummy rumbly though, you could make a case that Doryx would be worth a try. You'll have to decide if it's worth that 4000% price difference though, and there are other alternatives. While other antibiotics can cause stomach irritation as well, usually one can be found that a person can tolerate. Medications related to doxycycline, such as tetracycline or minocycline, can be used to treat acne, as well as antibiotics from other classes such as erythromycin and clindamycin. Of course there are plenty of other options as well, from antibiotics applied to the skin instead of taken orally, to topical creams and lotions such as Retin-A, or powerful drugs like isotretinoin for severe cases. Chances are very good that an effective acne treatment for you can be found without having to pay Doryx-like prices.

Chapter 15: Duac Gel

The Med

Back to the world of acne we go for this med, and if you've been reading the whole book to this point, a lot of what I have to say here will sound familiar. Duac is a combination of two active medications used in the treatment of pimples, clindamycin, an antibiotic, and benzoyl peroxide, which works as an anti-bacterial, and by removing excess skin oil and dead skin cells that can clog pores. Which sounds an awful lot like...

The Scam

...Acanya, the first med I talked about in this book. I'd like to think that in the world of medicine, a breakthrough in one area of medication therapy spurs many excited researchers to work to learn all about how a new med works, a frenzy of inquiry results, and the result is that many talented researchers put their own unique spin on what the breakthrough med has accomplished, and that's why we end up with many drugs that are similar to each other, each carving out its own niche where it is the best choice for a particular group of patients. I'd like to think that, but like I said earlier, Acanya is a rip off, and so is Duac. Both are a combination of an inexpensive topical antibiotic (clindamycin gel can be had for around $25), and an over the counter, readily available remedy (a tube of benzoyl peroxide will set you back around $5). Do the math and you'll see you can have a do it yourself version of Duac for around $30. So what is the retail price of a tube of Duac then?

$250, give or take a few dollars, which to be fair is less than Acanya. Also, Duac does at least use a strength of benzyol peroxide that is as strong as what you can buy on your own, not a strength that is actually weaker like Acanya. So I suppose you could make an argument that Duac is a relative bargain in the world of medication price gouging.

Neither one is a *good* deal though. As much as I'd like to think I lived in a different type of world, the only research involved in the creation of Duac and Acanya was in how to fleece consumers and insurance companies in ways to maximize revenue for their manufacturers, Stiefel Laboratories and Valeant Pharmaceuticals, respectively.

What To Do

It's the same game plan as with Acanya. If your doctor gives you a prescription for Duac, ask for one for clindamycin gel instead. Then buy yourself a tube of 5% benzoyl peroxide and a present for yourself with the money you'll save on your prescription bill and/or your insurance premiums.

Chapter 16: Duexis

The Med

Duexis is a combination of two different drugs, the pain reliever/anti-inflammatory ibuprofen, and the anti-ulcer/heartburn medication famotidine. Ibuprofen is among the most widely used drugs in the country, used by millions of people each day to combat everything from minor aches, pains, and fevers to full blown arthritis. These types of drugs are not without risk however. They are notoriously hard on the stomach, and can cause gastrointestinal bleeding that leads to an estimated 16,500 deaths every year. The idea behind Duexis is that combining ibuprofen with an acid-suppressing drug such as famotidine will help protect the stomach and lead to fewer adverse effects, and that idea is not a bad one. The problem is how this good idea is packaged and sold.

The Scam

Part of the reason both ibuprofen and famotidine are so popular is that they are not only effective, they are very cheap. A little online shopping and I located a bottle of 500 over the counter ibuprofen 200mg tablets for $6.98. A little more shopping and I found a bottle of 90 famotidine 10mg tablets available without a prescription for $7.88. Duexis takes the cheap out of equation though. While taking these two medicines together will protect your stomach, at over $150 a month, Duexis will do major damage to your wallet. If you're lucky enough to have prescription insurance coverage, the maker of Duexis, Horizon Pharma, does offer a "savings card" that allows you to shift part of this cost to your insurer, promising that you "may" pay as little as $20 for a Duexis prescription. The fine print, however, makes it clear that you may end up paying more. In any case, as you can see, Duexis is no bargain no matter how the "savings" card works out for you.

What To Do

There is no reason for Duexis to exist. None. Unless you're the kind of person who puts great value on being able to just swallow one tablet at a time. A do it yourself version of this product can be easily assembled without even so much as a trip to the doctor's office by just going to the pain reliever and antacid section of any drugstore. If you are under a physician's care though, and she determines that an ibuprofen and famotidine combination is for you, just have her write a separate prescription for each drug, as both can be had in prescription form for as little as $4 a month. That's $1700 in savings a year, which just might go a long way in easing whatever pain it is that ails you.

Chapter 17: Edluar

The Med

I'll admit that there is many a night I spend staring at the ceiling. That there is many a thing that can keep me from getting a good night's sleep. The latest plot twists on TV's "Mad Men," dreams about being chased by giant corn flakes, and other things that might be better not to write about here. The bottom line is, there are a lot of things that can keep me awake.

Evidently I am not alone. Sales of prescription sleep aids have gone through the roof in the last decade, with over 59 million prescriptions written in 2009 and sales totaling over $3 billion, the country's sleep troubles have become big business.

Edluar aims to capture part of that market with a unique twist. It is a formulation of the best selling sleep aid zolpidem, available for years under the brand name Ambien and now sold in inexpensive generic forms. Edluar claims to be different because it is a sublingual tablet, meaning you dissolve it under your tongue instead of washing it down with water the traditional tablet way.

The scam

Why is sublingual better? If you look over the official

Edluar web site, you will be hard pressed to find an answer. Edluar is "another option to help you fall asleep" it says, with "no need to get out of bed for a drink of water." Scouring the site from top to bottom, you will see no claims that Edluar is better, faster, or otherwise has any advantage over the regular zolpidem tablets millions of people have been using for years. You just dissolve it under your tongue, that's all. If getting out of bed for a drink of water is a major problem in your life that needs to be addressed, then I suppose Edluar could be the answer. And if it's worth it for you to pay $200 a month to solve this water problem of yours, then I guess you can stop reading now and ask your doctor if Edluar is right for you.

If you're looking for a bargain though, you can stick your insurance company with some of that cost through an Edluar "savings program" that claims you'll get your first month's prescription free and be paying $20 a month for four months afterwards. Read the fine print though, and you'll find you could be paying more.

But if that fine print says you're one of the lucky ones, before you get too excited about the big savings, I'll let you know that you can get a prescription for zolpidem tablets for around $15 a month. You will have to supply your own water though.

What To Do

If your doctor writes you a prescription for Edluar, ask her what advantage it has over regular zolpidem tablets. Other than it melts in your mouth, they won't be able to tell you one. It is the same med, in the same strength, that insomniacs have grown to know over the last 15 years. Believe me, if there were any advantage to this melting medicine, Meda Pharmaceuticals, Edluar's manufacturer, would not hesitate to let the world know. Instead, there is silence. They only claim that Edluar will save you a glass of water.

So if your doctor writes you a prescription for Edluar, kindly explain that you have a readily accessible water source, have them write for regular zolpidem instead, and enjoy an extra $2400 a year and the benefits of good hydration.

Chapter 18: Evoclin

The Med

We've talked about clindamycin and its use in the treatment of acne before. Part of the problem with pimples is that they are infected, which is why antibiotics like clindamycin have a role in their treatment. Over the years, clindamycin has evolved into a workhorse in the acne antibiotic field, becoming available for topical application as a gel, a lotion, and a solution. Evoclin continues this trend, as it is the first topical clindamycin foam.

The Scam

"How is Evoclin different from the clindamycin products that have come before?" you may be asking yourself if your doctor says it is right for you. "What are its advantages, the added benefits, the big distinction that makes Evoclin stand out?"

To which I would answer, "It's a foam. It's foamy."

Does it claim to work any better? Nope. It's just foamy.

Fewer side effects? Nope, I can't say that. It is foamy though.

Actually I'm not being quite fair here. According to the official package insert, Evoclin can be applied just once a day whereas the other forms of topical clindamycin are to be applied twice daily.

Evoclin's package insert also contains a warning that it is flammable, and that you should avoid fire, flame and/or smoking during and immediately following application. I'm not making that up. If you're a professional fire dancer or just a heavy smoker, then Evoclin probably isn't for you at any price.

If you decide you're in the market for Evoclin though, 50 grams costs $205.99 according to drugstore.com. Or you can get the 100 gram size for $322. If you're a bargain shopper though, you can indulge your foam fetish with a money saving generic that runs somewhere around $160, or $260 for 100 grams.

Or, you could buy one of the other forms of clindamycin, and spend anywhere from $16 to $45. I'll warn you though, you won't be getting any foam. Did I mention Evoclin is foamy?

What To Do

Unless you're just really, really, a foam fan, if your doctor hands you a prescription for Evoclin, ask her why. Unless she responds with a reason that convinces you a price difference of at least $120 is worth it, politely ask for a prescription for one of the other forms of topical clindamycin instead. There's no proof one works any better than the other, there's no proof one is any safer than the other, besides the open flame thing, but the other forms of clarithromycin are definitely superior at protecting your savings.

And if you really want to play with some foam, there's always shaving cream.

Chapter 19: Extina

The Med

Extina is a version of the topical antifungal medicine ketoconazole. While versions of ketoconazole are used for several types of fungal skin infections, Extina is officially indicated only for what is known as seborrhoeic dermatitis. Seborrheic dermatitis is an itchy, flaky condition of the scalp or other oil rich areas of the skin in which it is theorized the proliferation of microscopic yeast particles leads to an inflammatory reaction. Generic ketoconazole is sold as either a cream or a shampoo. Extina, however, is a ketoconazole foam.

The Scam

It would be easy to assume then, that since Extina is indicated only for seborrhoeic dermatitis, and since it is the only ketoconazole foam available, that Extina must have been shown to be more effective than other ketoconazole products. While I'd be willing to bet that the makers of Extina, Stiefel Laboratories, wouldn't mind very much if you believed that, there isn't a shred of evidence that it's true. The FDA, you see, can only reject a new drug application for one of two reasons, either 1) the drug doesn't work, or 2) it is too dangerous. Nowhere do you have to show your product is better than what is already on the market to get something approved, and nowhere does price come into consideration in the approval process. Stiefel Laboratories takes full advantage of this in the marketing of Extina. Only a single study is cited in the Extina professional labeling, and that study shows Extina is superior to a placebo foam. Dig a little deeper and you'll see that while that study showed 56 percent of patients met the criteria of "treatment success," so did 42 percent of the placebo foam users. So, when you're buying a can of Extina, what you're getting is a 14 percent chance that what you get will work better than a foam with no medicine at all.

And you'll pay around $200 for that chance. $400 if you decide to go for the large size. A generic foam is available for around $150, but before you decide how much of a bargain that is, let me tell you something.

Remember the ketoconazole shampoo that I mentioned earlier? The same med in the same strength as the foamy Extina, except in a form whose whole purpose is to be applied to a person's scalp? You can get a bottle of that for around $20. There's even an over the counter strength, Nizoral A-D, that you can buy without having to see your doctor.

What To Do

Let me be clear, I don't think ketoconazole is a bullshit drug. That 14% difference I mentioned earlier is definitely better than nothing and if my scalp were itching and flaking I would not hesitate to try some. I would not, however, pay $200 for the product, unless perhaps under the influence of a drug category I don't write about here. Unless you just really like foam, or unless your doctor can come up with a very compelling reason for foam, use the ketoconazole shampoo instead. Or even ketoconazole cream, which can be had for around $20 a tube.

Chapter 20: Fexmid

The Med

Fexmid is a brand name of the muscle relaxant cyclobenzaprine. Muscle spasms can often occur as a reaction to trauma or injury, and if they've ever happened to you, you don't need me to explain how painful they can be. Cyclobenzaprine has been sold under the brand name of Flexeril since 1977, and is also available in generic versions. It is widely used, cheap, and has over the years become a standard in the treatment of short term muscle spasms.

The Scam

Actually the "widely used" part of that description only applies to one strength of cyclobenzaprine, the 10 milligram tablets. It's also been sold in a 5mg strength for as long as I can remember, but 5mg prescriptions are relatively few and far between, usually only for the elderly, people with liver problems, or those who can't tolerate cyclobenzaprine's side effects, such as drowsiness. The fact that there is very little demand for any cyclobenzaprine other than a 10mg strength doesn't stop Shionogi Incorporated through, which markets Fexmid pretty much the same way you'd market an innovative new product.

It's not. Fexmid is simply 7.5 milligrams of cyclobenzaprine, and is sold for around $120 for thirty tablets. A prescription for the same number of 10mg generic cyclobenzaprine tablets can be had for around $10. So in case you missed it, with Fexmid you pay way more and actually get less. Something tells me though that they don't use that fact in their advertising slogans.

Don't get too excited that there is now a generic version of cyclobenzaprine 7.5mg either. It sells for around $100 for thirty tablets.

What To Do

It is possible that a 7.5mg dose of cyclobenzaprine might be right for some people. Like I said earlier, sometimes the med causes drowsiness that people find troubling. For that or some other reason it may be that your doctor thinks you just don't need as high a dose as most people. Make sure that's the case if you are given a prescription for Fexmid though, and that it isn't a situation where your doctor had a sales call from one of those ex college cheerleaders at some point. If it turns out that a 7.5mg dose really is the best plan for you, there's still an alternative. Have your doctor write a prescription for the 5mg tablets and take one and a half tablets as a dose. Your reward for a little pill splitting will be around an extra $90, and the satisfaction you outsmarted some very clever people in the business world.

Chapter 21: Glumetza

The Med

Glumetza is an extended-release version of metformin, a drug that has become a mainstay in the treatment of type 2 (formerly known as adult-onset) diabetes, which is responsible for the death of 60,000 Americans a year and is a contributing factor in 150,000 more. Diabetes is the leading cause of blindness in adults under 70 and leads to over 60,000 amputations annually. It is a leading cause of kidney disease and nerve damage, and also an incredible money making opportunity for Santarus, Inc.

The Scam

It may seem odd that a go-to drug used to treat one of the nation's leading killers would end up in a book about pharmacy rip-offs, and I know I promised in the introduction of this book not to go after mere extended-release formulations of established medicines. Glumetza, however, isn't just a regular tablet of metformin, and it claims to be more than just an extended release version of the med. Santarus explains in its marketing materials that Glumetza "uses advanced technology that delivers the type 2 diabetes medicine slowly and steadily over several hours. This delay in the release of metformin may result in fewer stomach-related side effects"

Hmm... well I say it may also result in your eyeballs catching fire, and there's as much proof for my claim as there is for Santarus'. While it's pretty clear Santarus wants you to think the chances of side effects with their product may be less than with regular metformin, I looked up and down and all around their pitch to the public and just could not find any hard numbers to back up their implication.

So I went to the official prescribing information. The mind-numbingly boring, small black-and-white text information required by the FDA to be produced and available to healthcare professionals. Here's what I found:

> "In the 24-week monotherapy trial comparing GLUMETZA to immediate release metformin, serious adverse reactions were reported in 3.6% (19/528) of the GLUMETZA treated patients compared to 2.9% (5/174) of the patients treated with immediate release metformin."

So...the only time Santarus actually comes up with any hard numbers involving stomach related side effects they say MORE people ran into problems than with regular metformin. This actually makes my total lack of eyeball combustion data look good by comparison. Maybe Santarus' marketing department should have worked that angle instead.

I'm kidding about the eyeball stuff of course, but I'm not kidding when I say Santarus tries to sell Glumetza as a version of metformin that might be easier on your stomach while providing numbers that imply it might actually be the exact opposite. If you think that's chutzpah, wait until you hear the price.

You or your insurance company will pay around $300 a month for Glumetza, compared to less than $15 for regular metformin tablets. That's close to $3400 a year for nothing but the suggestion from a drug company that their product "may" decrease gastrointestinal side effects, when the actual data in their prescribing information suggests otherwise.

What To Do

If your prescriber gives you a prescription for Glumetza ask him why. If your prescriber says it's because Glumetza causes fewer gastrointestinal side effects, ask him to prove it. He won't be able to. If, however, they can give you an explanation that justifies in your mind spending more than the average annual income of a citizen of the country of Moldova, then by all means, give the Glumetza a try. Otherwise, go with the regular metformin. Then if, and only if, you cannot tolerate any stomach-related side effects, and if taking smaller, more frequent doses of metformin doesn't make your tummy better, think about the theoretical, but completely unproven, Glumetza difference.

Chapter 22: Intermezzo

The Med

Some of you may have become confused when you saw the name of this entry, perhaps thinking you've accidentally gained access to a work on music theory. An intermezzo, after all, is known to many as a musical composition that connects acts of a larger work, such as a play or opera. In this case however, Intermezzo is another form of the drug zolpidem, the popular sleep aid most commonly sold under the brand name Ambien. The difference is that Intermezzo is a sublingual tablet, which means it's dissolved under your tongue instead of swallowed like a regular tablet. It's also available in different strengths, coming in 1.75 and 3.5 milligram versions, as opposed to Ambien's 5 and 10 mg.

The Scam

I've written about attempts to cash in on the huge sleep aid market before when I discussed Edluar and how its manufacturer, Meda Pharmaceuticals, tries to convince doctors and patients that the ability to dissolve a tablet under the tongue is worth a price increase of over tenfold. Intermezzo takes this idea one step further though, using its lower strength version of zolpidem to get an official indication "for the treatment of insomnia when a middle-of-the-night awakening is followed by difficulty returning to sleep." Remember what I told you earlier, as long as a drug company can show that a med works better than a placebo and is not overly dangerous, the FDA has to approve it. In case there's any doubt that the bar to distinguish a drug from that placebo is very, very, low, here are the results of a study as reported in Intermezzo's official labeling:

> *"Doses of 3.5 mg and 1.75 mg of Intermezzo significantly decreased both objective (by polysomnography) and subjective (patient-estimated) sleep latency after a scheduled middle of the night awakening as compared to placebo. The effect on sleep latency was similar for females receiving 1.75 mg of Intermezzo and males receiving 3.5 mg of Intermezzo."*

And how much was this decrease in the time it took for study subjects to get to sleep? Half an hour or ten seconds? We'll never know, because the official labeling never bothers to tell us.

There is one other study cited in the labeling, with similar, lackluster outcomes:

> *"Patients took study drug (3.5 mg of Intermezzo or placebo) on an as-needed basis, when they had difficulty returning to sleep after waking in the middle of the*

night, provided they had at least 4 hours time remaining in bed. Subjective (patient-estimated) time to fall back to sleep after middle-of-the-night awakening was significantly shorter for Intermezzo 3.5 mg compared to placebo."

Again, no hard numbers here, just study subjects reporting that they think they got to sleep quicker. Don't expect a Nobel Prize for this research anytime soon.

Of course it is intuitive that a low dose of zolpidem would help a person get back to sleep in the middle of the night without being overly drowsy in the morning. But science isn't about intuition and subjective subject-reported results. And there's nothing stopping you from snapping a regular 5 milligram zolpidem tablet in half and saving yourself $190 a month.

That's right, 30 days of this lower strength, waterless version of the Ambien so many already know and love will cost you around $200 at full retail price. Like so many of these rip-off meds though, there is a "savings card" program that claims to take $45 dollars off that total. Keep in mind though, a generic zolpidem prescription will cost around $15, no card required.

What To Do

Instead of letting Intermezzo serve as a connection

between the larger bills of your wallet and Purdue Pharma, ask your doctor for a 5mg prescription of regular zolpidem tablets instead. Snap them in half and report your subjective results to yourself in the morning.

Chapter 23: Jalyn

The Med

Jalyn is a combination of two drugs, dutasteride and tamsulosin, meant to counter one of the major design defects of the male body. Talk to me all you want about the majesty of the universe, the perfection of nature, the grand plan that rules us all, and I will counter with one simple fact: the prostate gland should never have been placed so that it wraps around the urethra. Anyone who looks at the simplest of diagrams of a man's reproductive system can see this. The urethra, you'll see, is the tube that carries urine from the bladder through the penis during its trip (hopefully) into a urinal or other sanitary appliance, and the prostate gland wraps right around it, like a hand loosely hanging onto a hose. The problem is, after a few decades of exposure to testosterone, the prostate starts to swell, which means it starts to squeeze on the tube that carries urine away from the bladder. Imagine that hand on a hose gripping tighter and tighter and you'll easily be able to figure out some of the most common symptoms of benign prostatic hyperplasia, or BPH.

- Urinary frequency, because the compressed urethra doesn't allow the bladder to completely empty.

- A constant feeling of having to pee, again because the bladder is never empty.

- Trouble starting to urinate because the urethra is partially blocked.

You get the idea. So the next time someone waxes poetic about the perfection of the human body, just remember, if the prostate gland had been designed by General Motors, someone like Ralph Nader would have forced them to recall it long ago.

The Scam

How many of you readers are college basketball fans, whipped into a frenzy each March with the onset of tournament madness? Those of you who are know that every year when the teams who'll play for the national championship are announced, there are always a few that are "on the bubble." Southwest Hillbilly State may have had an OK year, but everybody knows they really aren't of championship caliber. Still, teams are needed to fill the available number of slots, so the hillbillies get a crack at the title. When I was putting together my list of potential rip off drugs, I thought of Jalyn as kind of like that. It's definitely not the leader in the competition to fleece as much money as possible from your drug budget, but you still have to admire the effort, so I put them in the game. The scheme here is to put two medicines into one capsule in order to keep the patient away from a much lower priced alternative. Tamsulosin is available on its own, for around $20 a month. A drug very similar to dutasteride, which goes by the name of finasteride, is even more inexpensive. A month's supply can probably be had for around $10.

The price of Jalyn? Somewhere around $140 for thirty days. More than four times what most men would have to pay to get their prostate under control.

What To Do

Because Jalyn does use a medicine that is slightly different from finasteride, there is a chance that it will work better in some people than separate prescriptions for finasteride and tamsulosin. A small chance. If your doctor makes a move to give you a prescription for Jalyn, ask them if they think finasteride and tamsulosin would do the trick for you. Unless he gives you a good reason why they wouldn't, ask for prescriptions for finasteride and tamsulosin instead. Then enjoy an extra thousand dollars a year as well as your new role as the main character in so many prank phone calls: Mr. I.P. Freely.

Chapter 24: Keflex 750

The Med

Keflex is a brand name of the antibiotic cephalexin, and it is a workhorse of the medical world. Widely used to treat infections of the respiratory and urinary tract, ears, bone and skin, it is the most popular drug in its category (cephalosporins), as well as one of the most commonly prescribed medicines in the world, with over 25 million prescriptions filled each year in the United States alone. It is effective and inexpensive. Rather, I should say it's usually inexpensive.

The Scam

Since its introduction in 1967, Keflex has been available in 250 and 500 milligram strengths, as well as 125 and 250mg per teaspoonful liquid versions. This makes it easy to prescribe the drug in its official recommended dose, either 250mg every 6 hours or 500mg every 12 hours. For severe infections, the dose can be increased to up to 4000mg a day, which gave Shionogi Inc. an idea. Why not come out with a higher, 750mg strength and market it to be taken as two capsules twice a day? 3000mg a day will be at the upper end of the recommended dosage range for cephalexin, and the twice a day regimen will be easier for patients to follow than the commonly used four times a day.

I'll let you decide whether it was a desire for increased clinical effectiveness, patient convenience, or the $300 price tag for a prescription of Keflex 750 that motivated Shionogi to come up with this idea. But first I'll let you know that a course of the 250 or 500mg strengths would cost you around $15.

What To Do

The thing is, there's nothing special or different about Keflex 750. Shionogi isn't trying the old "extended release" or "slightly different version that qualifies for a new patent" tricks. It's just more of the same medicine crammed into a capsule. And if you do a little math, you'll soon notice it's not hard at all to replicate what they've done. They want you to put 750mg of cephalexin in your stomach by taking one of their capsules, but there's no reason you can't put 750mg of cephalexin in your stomach by taking three 250mg capsules, and saving yourself over $200 in the process.

So, if your doctor wants to prescribe Keflex 750, and the increased trouble of taking three capsules instead of one is something you're willing to deal with, ask her for a prescription for the 250mg instead. The money you save at the pharmacy counter should more than make up for whatever you have to give your local utility for the extra water to get a few more capsules down.

Chapter 25: Latisse

The Med

When I first heard of Latisse, it made me question my medical knowledge. Later, as I learned more, it made me question my sexuality. Latisse, you see, is the first prescription eye drop to treat hypotrichosis, which sounds scary and serious. My first thought was maybe hypotrichosis was the fancy medical name for African River Blindness or some other dreadful sight threatening condition. But when I looked it up I learned that scary sounding hypotrichosis is actually:

"inadequate or not enough eyelashes"

This was a problem? I started a search for the signs and symptoms of this condition. I wondered what the prognosis was for sufferers. Allergan, the maker of Latisse, seemed very excited about it, so I figured this new treatment must be some type of revolutionary medical breakthrough. But after I dug into things for awhile, I learned that most "patients" that were to come to me with prescriptions for Latisse simply wanted to be sexier.

That was a surprise to me, because I'm pretty sure I've never once said to myself, or heard anyone else ever say anything like, "Whoa!! Check out her eyelashes!!"

I've never once had eyelashes figure into a dating decision or complimented a woman on hers a single time. Maybe eyelashes play a role in human sexuality that I was completely unaware of. Maybe I'm some sort of prude.

The Scam

Or maybe Allergan is taking advantage of the extreme shallowness that prevails in modern society. Latisse is nothing new. It is simply a repackaging of the anti-glaucoma medicine Lumigan. The people at Allergan noticed that glaucoma sufferers using their product sometimes grew thicker eyelashes, so they put it in a different box and pretended it was something new. It is not. It is the same stuff, in the same strength, with the same side effects, including the risk that it may change the color of your eyes to brown. The only difference is Latisse is packaged with a supply of little brushes that make applying it to your lashes easier. Let me repeat this to be clear: there is no difference between Latisse and Lumigan other than the name on the box.

If you decide that sexy eyelashes are what you want though, and you really desire the little brushes to help you put on your Lumig....er....Latisse, be ready to pay around $110 a month.

What To Do

Pick up a book, because a smart woman is the sexiest of them all. Why do you think librarians and nurses play such prominent roles in fantasy lives? While you're in that book maybe you'll learn that African River Blindness has taken the sight of over 300,000 people even though it can be treated for only a few dollars. Maybe then you'll be at the bar talking about the unfairness of it all and you'll sweep a socially conscious hunk of a man right off his feet. Or, at the very least, you could join a gym, and develop the parts of your body a shallow man-pig would actually be attracted to while doing wonders to improve your overall health.

Because Latisse, while marketed for the treatment of hypotrichosis, is far more effective in curing "more money than brains" syndrome.

Chapter 26: Luxiq

The Med

Luxiq is a form of the topical steroid betamethasone, a medicine that has been around for decades and is used to treat itchy, inflammatory skin conditions and rashes. The Luxiq difference? Unlike the creams, ointments, and lotions doctors, pharmacists, and patients have gotten used to over the years, Luxiq is a betamethasone foam.

The Scam

Again with the foam. Some of you might be reminded here of Extina, the antifungal foam we talked about earlier, and with good reason. Just like with Extina, Luxiq makes no claims to be better, safer, or otherwise have any advantage over any other forms of betamethasone other than being...foamy.

I probably should backtrack a little before I say there is no advantage of foamy betamethasone versus betamethasone in a lotion or cream. A bottle of Luxiq will set you or your insurance company back around $200, while a bottle of betamethasone lotion can be had for about $70. If you decide you're OK with betamethasone in a cream form, you'll probably pay less than $20.

As you can see, there is a big advantage to be had for using Luxiq- for its manufacturer, Stiefel Laboratories. Stiefel is also the company behind Extina, and says on its website that it employs scientists who "are dedicated to the advancement of skin research and use state-of-the-art human skin models to study drug delivery, efficacy and safety in pursuit of innovative dermatological products."

Which means that from now on, whenever I hear the word "innovative" I'll think "foam." Because evidently taking old, effective, cheap drugs and turning them into expensive foams seems to be what passes for state of the art research in at least one company. Because as you'll see later, the subject of Stiefel and their innovative foams will come up again.

What To Do

Again, just like with Extina, if you really like foam, you really don't have to do anything. It's not like Luxiq is ineffective, and if you just enjoy knowing your medicine has little air pockets dispersed throughout, then by all means, it's a free country. Keep in mind though, that Luxiq is far from free. Its official indication is to treat psoriasis of the scalp, and if that's what your doctor is using it for, than a betamethasone lotion would probably be the easiest alternative to use. If your doc is using Luxiq "off label" for another type of skin condition though, or if you decide that you're OK with a cream or ointment, keep in mind that those are usually even more economical options than the lotion. Either way, you'll have an extra hundred dollars or so in your pocket to buy something that is truly innovative.

Chapter 27: Magnacet

The Med

Everybody hurts, and because of that pain is big business for pharmaceutical companies. More than 244 million prescriptions were written for narcotic painkillers in 2010, which, according to the Centers for Disease Control and Prevention, was enough to keep every American adult medicated around the clock for a month. There is Vicodin, Vicodin ES and Vicodin HP. There is Tylenol with Codeine, Norco, Lorcet and Lortab, which by the way, comes in a liquid form, making it a bit of an oxymoron. These and dozens of other products stand ready to ease the pain that troubles you. The king of the drugstore narcotics however, is a drug by the name of oxycodone. Most famous as the extended release form OxyContin, this powerful pain reliever has become notorious as "hillbilly heroin," or "the crack of the countryside" as its abuse has cut a swath of devastation and destruction through rural communities. Used properly though, oxycodone is a valuable tool in the treatment of serious pain. Magnacet combines oxycodone with a dose of acetaminophen, the over the counter pain reliever better known by the brand name Tylenol, which provides the benefits of an additional pain med while cutting down on oxycodone's abuse potential.

The Scam

The thing is, Shionogi Incorporated, manufacturer of Magnacet, wasn't the first company to think of this idea. Oxycodone and acetaminophen combinations have been around for years, sold under brand names such as Percocet and Tylox and now available as cheap as dirt generics. Magnacet is just different enough however, using a slightly different strength of acetaminophen, that if your doctor writes the word "Magnacet" on a prescription, a pharmacy cannot give you one of the cheap generics. They are bound to give you Magnacet and Magnacet only.

What does that mean for you? Get a prescription for a hundred Magnacet tablets in the 5/400 strength and you or your insurance company will be out around $600. Get a prescription for Percocet 5/325, the oxycodone/acetaminophen combination we've all grown to know and love over the years, and it'll probably cost you $30 or less. I'm not kidding you. That's $550 for 75 milligrams of Tylenol. That's over seven dollars a milligram. That's the Magnacet difference.

What To Do

Unless you are a stockholder of Shionogi Incorporated, the kind of person who just likes the shape of Magnacet tablets so much it's worth a few hundred dollars a month to look at them, or maybe are in some sort of contest to see how much money you can spend, if your doctor hands you a prescription for Magnacet, ask her for one for Percocet instead. Your pain will be just as eased and your wallet will be far fatter.

Chapter 28: Makena

The Med

Makena is a brand name for an injectable version of the drug hydroxyprogesterone, which is used to reduce the risk of premature birth in women with a history of delivering early. Its manufacturer, KV Pharmaceutical, says Makena "is the first and only FDA approved medication that helps reduce risk for another preterm birth." No one could argue that premature birth isn't a serious issue, and if there is only one FDA approved medication to prevent it, how could that med possibly end up in a book about rip-off drugs? Read on.

The Scam

The statement that Makena is "the first and only FDA approved medication that helps reduce risk of another preterm birth" is true as far as it goes. But when KV won that approval in 2011, there was nothing new about hydroxyprogesterone. It originally hit pharmacy shelves in 1956 and was eventually pulled from the market as it fell out of favor among doctors as a treatment for uterine cancer or hormonal problems.

Some scientists suspected though, that the drug might have value in preventing premature birth, and in 2003, a study showed they were right. Doctors started writing prescriptions for injectable hydroxyprogesterone, which were filled by pharmacists who compounded the drug themselves, usually for around 10 to 20 dollars a dose. It was a cheap and effective way to prevent a devastating medical problem. Everybody wins.

Enter KV Pharmaceutical.

After the company obtained official FDA approval to market Makena, they almost immediately claimed they now had exclusive rights to sell the drug, and that any version individually compounded in a pharmacy was now illegal. Cease and desist letters were sent out, and KV Pharmaceutical went ahead with plans to become the sole distributor of hydroxyprogesterone.

The price they set? $1500 a dose. And since the injection must be given every week, an entire course of therapy could cost upwards of $30,000. After a public outcry, KV lowered the price by over 50% to $690 a week, still over 30 times what compounding pharmacies were charging.

By the way, that 2003 study that showed hydroxyprogesterone to be effective? It was funded by the National Institutes of Health, which means KV Pharmaceutical tried to use your tax dollars to secure a lucrative monopoly for itself.

The FDA however, stepped in and said it would not take enforcement action against individual pharmacies that continued to compound hydroxyprogesterone, putting a crimp in KV Pharmaceutical's profit scheme.

As of this writing, a lawsuit to reverse the FDA's decision has been thrown out, and KV has filed for Chapter 11 bankruptcy protection.

What To Do

As it stands now, hydroxyprogesterone is available both from compounding pharmacies and as KV's branded Makena, which the company claims "is manufactured in a facility that complies with FDA's Good Manufacturing Practices (GMPs)." They then draw a contrast to drugs made by compounding pharmacies, which they say "may present risks to patients because they have not been evaluated for safety and effectiveness by FDA, or if they have been improperly compounded." The implication is clear, when you pay the price for brand name Mankana, you are paying for quality.

Some things to keep in mind as you make your decision though, in 2009 KV recalled most of the products it manufactured after the FDA found "the company had significant GMP violations." Also, as of this writing, another product made by KV, a vaginal antibiotic cream called Clindesse, is not available due to a nationwide recall "because it may have been manufactured under conditions that did not sufficiently comply with current Good Manufacturing Practices."

Of course many of you are also probably familiar with the case of the New England Compounding Center. A compounding "pharmacy" that sold contaminated injectable products responsible for a nationwide outbreak of fungal meningitis that has killed, as of this writing, 44 people. It's important to know though, that the New England Compounding Center wasn't a pharmacy in the sense you or I recognize the word. You could not walk in and have a prescription filled, buy some aspirin, or talk to the pharmacist about your medication questions. Rather, NECC stretched the legal definition of the word pharmacy and used the fact that a pharmacist is legally entitled to compound individual prescriptions for individual patients as a loophole to become in essence a small-scale unregulated pharmaceutical factory. There is a world of difference between the individual pharmacist working behind the counter of their own store to make a prescription on the order of your local doctor and places like NECC.

In the end it's your decision. Base it on who you trust more, your local compounding pharmacy, or KV Pharmaceutical.

Chapter 29: Moxatag

The Med

I remember hearing a story in pharmacy school that has stuck with me ever since. My professor was talking about the dawn of the age of antibiotics and how they completely revolutionized the world of medicine. Penicillin in particular he said, was so valuable and so rare during World War II that when it was given to soldiers their urine would be saved so the drug could be crystallized out and used again. I never bothered to find out if that was really true, because if it wasn't it would ruin a great tale. It is a fact though that penicillin was at one time incredibly valuable and it and its related medicines did indeed change healthcare forever.

Moxatag is an extended-release version of the antibiotic amoxicillin, a close relative of penicillin and probably the most widely used workhorse in the antibiotic world. Amoxicillin is prescribed for everything from inner ear infections to sinusitis, pneumonia to bronchitis to tonsillitis and more. It can even have a role to play in the treatment of stomach ulcers. It's incredibly valuable and happily inexpensive - most of the time.

The Scam

I know I said in the introduction to this book that I wouldn't cover "extended release" scams. That while they are often simply an excuse for a drug company to milk extra revenue out of old product by pretending it's something new, you could make an argument that there is some benefit to be had in not having to take a medicine as often. It's an argument that Shionogi Incorporated makes on the Moxatag website, with the words "Keep it simple" being front and center so they'll be the first ones you'll see.

It's just that there's a little more to this extended release plot than most others. Moxatag is a 775 milligram, once a day tablet, and its prescribing information says it is to be used for tonsillitis and/or pharyngitis.

That's 775 milligrams once a day. Now stick with me here, because the normal adult doing for tonsillitis/pharyngitis using regular amoxicillin is 250 to 500mg three times a day. Alternately, a prescriber can also go with a twice a day dose of 500 or 875mg. Do the math and you'll see that the accepted dosage range to treat tonsillitis and or pharyngitis is anywhere from 750 to 1,750 milligrams a day.

A once a day Moxatag regimen fits into that dose range. Barely. And will cost around $150 dollars. A ten day course of twice a day 875mg tablets on the other hand, will probably run you around $15. With Moxatag, you pay way more and get a lot less. Shionogi does offer a "copay card" however, that, if you meet the terms and conditions, might allow you to get less and stick your insurance company with the added cost.

I guess I can see now why Shionogi's marketing people decided to play up the "Keep it simple" angle.

What To Do

Like I said earlier, there might be a situation where you feel a once a day antibiotic is the answer. Maybe you're a caregiver for a patient with swallowing difficulties or maybe you just don't trust yourself to remember to take a dose of medicine more than once a day. If that's the case, then by all means Moxatag might be the answer. Just remember there is a big price to pay for the Moxatag difference. If you're not married to the once a day idea though, ask your prescriber for a prescription for regular amoxicillin instead. You could buy yourself some sort of pill reminder alarm with the money you save and still come out way ahead.

Chapter 30: Niravam

The Med

We live in anxious times, or at least that would be a safe assumption based on our medication use. Benzodiazepines, a group of drugs used, among other things, to treat anxiety and panic disorder, have been flying off pharmacy shelves for almost 50 years, and alprazolam is the most popular member of this extremely popular group. Sold most commonly under the brand name Xanax, close to 50 million prescriptions were written for alprazolam alone in 2011. Niravam was brought to market in 2005 as a sublingual version of alprazolam.

The Scam

When I first heard of Niravam tablets I thought they would be a wonderful solution to a very insignificant problem. A sublingual tablet is simply one that dissolves under the tongue you see, and we already referred to generic Xanax tablets as "rice grains" around the pharmacy. A sublingual tablet is no more powerful than a regular tablet, no more effective, and has no fewer side effects. It just dissolves under the tongue instead of being swallowed. That would be great if you had trouble swallowing a regular tablet, but we called the regular alprazolams "rice grains" for a reason. There just aren't that many people who wouldn't be able to swallow one, and for those few people, there's nothing to stop them from crushing, cutting, chewing, grinding, or doing anything they have to do to get it down.

Jazz Pharmaceuticals, the manufacturer of Niravam, might make an argument that a sublingual tablet puts medicine into your bloodstream faster. We don't really know though, as they have next to nothing to say about their product on the company's website. Keep in mind though, there is nothing stopping you from grinding up a regular alprazolam tablet and holding the powder under your tongue. If you'd rather save yourself a little work though, and go the Niravam route, just know that it'll cost you.

How much? Thirty tablets of the most common strength of regular alprazolam tablets can easily be had for under ten dollars. Even though there is now a generic version of the sublingual Niravam, a prescription for 30 tablets of the same strength will most likely cost around $70.

It's enough to make a person hyperventilate.

What To Do

Unless you really just can't swallow a pill under any circumstances, or unless a few minutes difference to onset of action are critical and you are unable or unwilling to crush or chew a regular tablet, don't bother with Niravam. It is the same medicine in the same strength as a regular alprazolam tablet. It is just as effective and carries the same side effect profile, it just costs ten times as much. Have your doctor write a prescription for the regular alprazolam, and use the extra money in your wallet to buy yourself some peace of mind.

Chapter 31: Olux-E

The Med

Olux is a version of the potent corticosteroid clobetasol. Used topically to treat itching and swelling of the skin, clobetasol is usually reserved for the most serious conditions, such as plaque psoriasis or severe eczema, or for places on the body where the skin is thickest, such as the palms and bottom of the feet. Clobetasol generally isn't used for more than three weeks at a time, due to the possibility of side effects that can occur when the body absorbs too much of a steroid, such as weight gain, tiredness, muscle weakness, depression, and high blood pressure.

The Scam

Earlier in the book I wrote about Luxiq, another corticosteroid made by Stiefel Laboratories, and before that I wrote about the foamy product Extina, so a reader could be forgiven if they think I am about to repeat myself. Like Luxiq, Olux-E is a foamy version of a topical med also available in various cream, ointment, and lotions. Like Luxiq, Olux-E is the same drug doctors and pharmacists have become familiar with over the course of years, just in a foam. And like Luxiq, there's nothing necessarily wrong with getting a foamy steroid, but if that's what you decide you want to do, you will pay dearly for the privilege. A bottle of the smallest size of Olux-E will cost you somewhere around $250. If you want to go large, it'll be more like $480.

If that price makes you want to do some bargain hunting, you can do better. A generic version of Olux-E sells for around $130.

But wait, you can do even better. Clobetasol is also available as a solution that sells for around $30. Or at its most economical, as a cream that goes for less than $15. To you and me, a foam may just be a fluffy semi-liquid, but to the people at Stiefel Labs, a foam is evidently pure gold.

What To Do

Someone in sales would be likely to say the main advantage of a foam is in applying it to a place such as the scalp, where you can just rub it in and have little residue left behind. It is an advantage shared with gels and especially lotions though, and clobetasol comes in both forms that are far easier on your pocketbook. It could be well worth it to ask your prescriber for one of these instead of a prescription for Olux-E. If your problem isn't in a hairy place, or if you're just willing to put up with a cream, it could be worth talking to your prescriber about that as well. Olux-E is a good option for those that have a need for conspicuous consumption though, as well as people who suffer from fat wallet syndrome. As always though, the final choice is up to you.

Chapter 32: Oracea

The Med

I always saw Rudolph the Red Nosed Reindeer as the patron saint of rosacea sufferers. Rudolph suffered gallantly with his condition, the redness, the swelling, the mother of all pustules there on the end of his face. He endured the taunts and ostracization of his peers with courage and dignity. I have to be honest, I wouldn't have been nearly as gracious as Rudolph was when Santa came looking for help. I would have told Santa to stick it.

Fortunately for Rudolph and the other 16 million Americans with this inflammatory skin condition, today there are several good treatment options available. Among the most popular is the antibiotic doxycycline, and Oracea is a low dose version of the drug meant specifically for the treatment of rosacea. Just think, if Santa had known a good veterinarian or dermatologist, there's a chance a generation of children would have been scarred by an empty Christmas they would have never been able to forget.

The Scam

The only thing new about Oracea is the amount of drug per capsule, 40 mg as opposed to the 50 and 100 mg strengths that have been available for generations. Galderma claims in its advertising that Oracea is "not an antibiotic," because at the low dose found in the product, it works by taking advantage solely of anti-inflammatory properties of doxycycline, and blood levels never get high enough to actually have any antimicrobial effect. This is like saying if you take a tiny dose of strychnine than it is not a poison. Any clinical differences between a 40 mg dose or Oracea and a 50 mg dose of traditional doxycycline are unproven.

You'll pay over $400 for a month's worth of oracea though, as opposed to around $15 for doxycycline 50 mg capsules. That's 385 more dollars for 20 percent less drug.

Let's say you're the careful type though, and like the fact that 40 mg of doxycycline a day can treat your rosacea without killing off any bacteria. Is there any alternative to forking over big bucks? Yes. There is a 20 mg doxycycline tablet on the market, and while at around $50 a month it is more pricey than some of your other options, you'll still have an extra $4,200 in your pocket at the end of a year as opposed to going the Oracea route.

Galderma, Oracea's manufacturer, does offer a "savings card" that promises that if you have insurance and meet the program's conditions, you'll pay no more than $25 a month. Look closely though, and you'll see that the "savings card" is good for only a maximum benefit of $325. With today's high-deductible and high-copay insurance plans, that's a benefit you could go through very quickly. Read the fine print of both the "savings card" offer and your insurance policy before you sign up.

What To Do

I can't think of a single reason for Oracea to exist. It is incredibly overpriced and the only advantage its maker claims is that it maintains blood levels low enough to not have an antimicrobial effect. That may or may not be significant. Remember, you are still exposing bacteria long term to a chemical designed to kill them, and there is no proof that low-dose, long term exposure to doxycycline leads to fewer problems with bugs becoming antibiotic resistant. If I were battling a case of rosacea and my doctor wanted to use doxycycline, I would ask for a 50 mg prescription and save myself some big bucks. If you think there might be something to Galderma's low dose argument though, ask for the 20 mg tablets and save yourself some medium bucks.

Let's not tell Rudolph though. Just in case this Christmas Eve is another foggy one.

Chapter 33: Paxil CR

The Med

Paxil CR is a version of the extremely popular prescription drug paroxetine. Originally brought to market as an antidepressant in 1992, the med has since gained indications for use in the treatment of obsessive-compulsive, panic, social anxiety, posttraumatic stress and generalized anxiety disorders, and is consistently on any list of best selling prescription products in the country. It hasn't been a drug without controversy though, as there have been lawsuits that accused GlaxoSmithKline (GSK), the maker of both the original form of Paxil as well as Paxil CR, of downplaying paroxetine's side effect profile, the risk of suicide in pediatric patients using the drug, and hiding unfavorable research information about the drug. Despite this though, there is a general consensus that paroxetine has an important role to play in the treatment of mental health disorders, and that for millions of patients, the benefits of the medicine will outweigh the risks. Paroxetine is not the scam here, it's when we add the letters "CR" to the end that the problem happens.

The Scam

The "CR" scam may again leave some of you confused. Here I go again talking about a "CR" type med when I said in the introduction to this book that I wouldn't get into the old "continuous release" trick. Because even though drug companies do use "CR," "ER", "XR" and similar forms of drugs as revenue enhancers, you can argue that there is some benefit in having to take a medication less often.

I've said this a lot now, but there are a lot of times when drug companies have taken the "CR" trick the extra mile.

The original Paxil for instance, is taken once a day, which is the exact same number of times Paxil CR is taken per day. What gives? What possible advantage could there be to a continuous release product that is taken on the same dosage schedule?

GSK tried to claim that despite the "CR" at the end of its name, this new Paxil's advantage wasn't in the number of times it is taken, but rather, that it would have fewer side effects. By delaying the release of drug until the pill was past the stomach and into the intestine by using a controlled release mechanism, GSK implied that Paxil CR would cut down on paroxetine's notorious tendency to cause nausea in patients taking it.

The problem is that implication is never the foundation of sound science. Let's look at the numbers.

I went through the official prescribing information and found six studies that compared the rates of nausea reported in patients taking Paxil against those who were assigned to take a placebo. Here's what I found:

Study	% Of Patients With Nausea Reported on Paxil	% Of Patients With Nausea Reported on Placebo
1	26	9
2	23	10
3	23	17
4	25	7
5	20	5
6	19	8

As you can see, nausea certainly seems to be a problem with paroxetine therapy. You could see why a company might be looking for ways to counter it, as there's probably a lot of money to be made from people who would rather not feel like they have to throw up.

Now let's see how well Paxil CR solves the problem. I found five studies in its prescribing info:

Study	% Of Patients With Nausea Reported on Paxil CR	% Of Patients With Nausea Reported on Placebo
1	22	10
2	23	17
3	22	6
4	17	7
5	18	2

I think, looking at these numbers closely, you can see why I never found any studies that directly compared Paxil vs. Paxil CR. Using GSK's own numbers, it would seem you can pay around $10 a month for the generic version of regular Paxil, and run about a one in four risk that you'll end up feeling nauseous, or, you can try Paxil CR, and have your nausea chances go to roughly... one in four.

You'll also pay around $85 a month for this exact same risk. Even though Paxil CR now comes in its own generic form. My guess is that the "CR" in Paxil's case really stood for "continuing revenue."

What To Do

Unless you've had a problem with nausea while taking paroxetine, I can't think of any reason at all to be on

Paxil CR. If you are having problems with your stomach on Paxil, a different drug will be more likely to solve the problem than trying Paxil CR. Unless your prescriber can make a very good case otherwise, do your wallet a favor and stick with regular Paxil. Your stomach probably won't know the difference.

Chapter 34: Pexeva

The Med

Pexeva is yet another version of paroxetine, the same drug as the Paxil CR we just finished talking about. It's not a sustained release form though, and neither is it any of the other tricks so often employed by the pharmaceutical industry to separate a patient from their money. It doesn't come in a different package telling you it's for a different indication. It's not orally disintegrating. It's not even foamy. Pexeva is different only because it's a different salt form of the active drug. Pexeva is chemically paroxetine *mesylate*, while the original version of paroxetine, Paxil, is paroxetine *hydrochloride*. What does this mean? To make a long story short, when you take a salt into your body, it dissolves into separate sets of ions. Common table salt, for example, will dissolve into sodium ions and chloride ions. When you take a tablet of Paxil, it will dissolve into paroxetine ions and chloride ions, and Pexeva will dissolve into paroxetine and mesylate ions.

The Scam

Your body, however, is only interested in the paroxetine. It couldn't care less about what it's attached to. Hooking it up with mesylate as opposed to chloride doesn't make Pexeva any more or less effective. It also doesn't make it any safer nor more dangerous. You would be hard pressed to find any difference at all in how Pexeva works as opposed to Paxil, and Noven Therapeutics, Pexeva's manufacturer, doesn't even try.

Why did they even bother taking the time and trouble to come out with a drug that offers no advantage to an already long established and widely used medicine? Because the slight difference in chemistry between Pexeva and Paxil is just enough to allow Pexeva to be marketed as a new product. If your doctor writes a prescription for Pexeva, it cannot be filled with Paxil or one of its generic forms.

Pexeva, however will cost you or your insurer around $200 a month, while a prescription filled for a month's worth of generic Paxil shouldn't cost you any more than $10. That's the difference that makes all of Noven Therapeutic's time and trouble worthwhile, even after they offer you a $50 "savings" card from their website.

What To Do

I once got an email a few years back after I wrote an article about Pexeva:

> *"I just wanted to thank you immensely for the post you did concerning idiotic doctors who give Pexeva prescriptions instead of paroxetine. My husband was*

diagnosed as bipolar about a year ago. We have been in terrible financial condition, in large part to his inability to work because of his mental issues. After years of discussion, I finally got him to see a doctor about it. He was diagnosed using the same damn checklist I found online years before and the doctor prescribed Pexeva. It was like a miracle - he was under control for the first time in a long time. The only problem was that his prescription cost about $200 a month (he's uninsured), and it was very hard to scrape the money together to pay for it.

Imagine my surprise when googling around about a generic alternative, I found your post. THANK YOU SO MUCH! Our dumbass doctor didn't believe there was a generic Pexeva (amazing!!) so I printed your post and enlightened him. Incredibly, it took some arm-twisting to get the damn paroxetine prescription from him, but we got it. $4 freaking dollars a month at any Wal-Mart or Kroger's; hell of a difference from $200 a month. Honestly, we can now pay the electric bill thanks to you!!!

It made me feel good to know I had won a small victory in the fight against the large breasts of pharmaceutical sales reps, and that I had literally brought some light into the world. You too can win a victory over breast tissue. If you are given a prescription for Pexeva, ask your prescriber why they chose it over Paxil, and listen very carefully to the answer. Then email me at dstan93940@gmail.com and let me know what your prescriber said, as I am very interested in what the sales reps are telling prescribers in order to move this stuff. Unless the answer you hear is very compelling, which I have a feeling it won't be, ask them to write you a prescription for paroxetine instead, and enjoy being able to leave the lights on a little longer.

Chapter 35:
Poly-Vi-Flor/Tri-Vi-Flor

The Med

At one time I would have put the Poly and Tri-Vi-Flor line of products on any list of the most boring prescription medications ever. Simply vitamin and fluoride supplements, ("Poly" is a more complete vitamin formula, while "Tri" has only vitamins A, C, and D) they require a prescription only to ensure a child doesn't get too high of a fluoride dose, which can damage the very teeth your doctor or dentist are looking to protect. Ho hum, just vitamins and fluoride. They're cheap products whose purpose is to keep a healthy body running at peak efficiency that can be sold at cheap prices and still provide a nice profit for both manufacturer and retailer. Everybody wins! How could you possibly improve on this boring situation?

The Scam

Well, if you're Zylera Pharmaceuticals, the improvement potential here is obvious. Buy the boring Poly and Tri-Vi-Flor names, change the formula around to make it (seem) sexier, and transform the product into a cheap med than can be sold at an expensive price.

The key to Poly and Tri-Vi-Flor's newfound sexy self is Metafolin, a patented form of folate, a basic B vitamin that has been available forever, most commonly in the form of folic acid. What makes Metafolin special? Basically the pre-digestion difference. When a person takes folic acid, some basic metabolism takes place that eventually changes it around to L-methylfolate, the form that is actually used by the body. There's nothing special or unique about this process. A good part, if not the majority, of vitamins, minerals, medications and other building blocks of your body are metabolized like this into their useful form. If that weren't the case, your liver would be out of a job and on the unemployment line. What patent holder Merck was able to do was figure out how to make the active form of folic acid synthetically and then fill out the paperwork that allowed them to be the only ones allowed to sell it. So another way to think of Metafolin is as pre-digested folic acid, which doesn't seem nearly as sexy as the advertising descriptions I've read from Merck.

If you're still turned on though, then the new Poly or Tri-Vi-Flor may just be for you. The addition of Metafolin is the difference between the sexy stuff and the Plain Jane Poly or Tri-Vi-Flor your doctor most likely meant to prescribe. If a prescriber writes the words "Poly-Vi-Flor" or "Tri-Vi-Flor" on a prescription pad these days though, the pre-digested version is what a pharmacist is legally required to give you. And you or your insurance company will pay around $200 a month for the privilege of having some digestion done for you at a factory instead of in your liver or other organs.

I'm starting to regret ever using the word "sexy" here.

What To Do

The original, boring, Poly and Tri-Vi-Flor formulas that took care of the nutritional and fluoridation needs of generations of Americans are still available, and you can get them for under $15 dollars a month. Like I said though, the key is to avoid actually getting a prescription for Poly or Tri-Vi-Flor. You can do this by having your prescriber just write something like "multivitamins with fluoride" "tri-vitamins with fluoride" or even "Poly-Vi-Flor, old formula" on your prescription. You won't get the benefits of having some of your digestion done for you ahead of time, but you will have an extra $2200 a year in your pocket, with which I'm betting you can buy a whole lot of sexy.

Chapter 36: Renova

The Med

Oh the ravages of time. This I can promise you dear reader, no matter how strong and able you are this day, no matter how ravishing your looks or sharp your brain, even if you are now at an apex of human development never before reached by our species, the blueprints of your demise have already been laid. One day, and sooner than you may think, you will start to slow, bit by bit. You will tire just a little sooner than you used to, and then a little sooner than that. Parts of your body will sink and sag, grow soft and turn to flab. You can delay but not stop this I am afraid to tell you. Every person on this planet, each of us without exception, suffers from one common malady. We are all getting old. Renova, however, promises help with one sign of this condition. If you need assistance in the mitigation of fine facial wrinkles, then Renova, a topical version of the drug tretinoin, might just be a type of time machine in a tube you are looking for.

The Scam

A tube of tretinoin however, is far from a new thing. Some of you may remember me sharing earlier how tretinoin was my ticket out of the world of teenage acne. But, you may be thinking, aren't we talking about wrinkles now, and aren't those two different conditions? Yes we are, and they are, and that's exactly how the people at Valeant Pharmaceuticals want you to think.

Tretinoin originally came to market as a product called Retin-A, which was marketed exclusively as an acne treatment and is available in 0.01, 0.025, 0.05, and 0.1 percent strengths. By the time widespread use revealed that tretinoin may be effective in reducing facial wrinkles though, Ortho pharmaceuticals was close to losing its patent on the product, and decided doing formal studies on a medicine that was about to face generic competition wouldn't be cost effective. Doctors began to prescribe tretinoin "off label" for wrinkle reduction, the generics came out, the price went down, and that seemed to be that.

Until someone at Valeant decided there was still some profit potential here. Renova came out as a 0.02% product, and a study was done showing that this 0.02% strength was more effective in reducing wrinkles than a placebo. So while it may stand to reason and appeal to common sense that you could use any tretinoin strength to treat wrinkles, technically, the people at Valeant can say theirs is the only product proven to work.

The price for a tube? Somewhere in the neighborhood of $200. While a tube of the 0.025% tretinoin cream can be had for around $40. Think that over while you remember the standard answer from the pharmaceutical industry whenever they are asked why prescriptions are so expensive. Because of all the money that goes into the research necessary in bringing a new product to market they will say.

What To Do

Unless you're the type of person who feels that the effect of a 0.005% reduction of topical tretinoin dose is a scientific question whose answer is really worthy of your dollars, if your prescriber hands you a prescription for Renova, ask for the 0.025% tretinoin instead. True, you will be going out on an unpaved scientific trail, but maybe with the $1900 you save a year, you can contribute a little to a study that shows the regular tretinoin works just fine.

Chapter 37: Reprexain

The Med

There is pain and suffering in this world, and I don't think anyone with the slightest bit of awareness can deny this. I hurt, you hurt, as those great philosophers of song R.E.M. once noted, "Everybody Hurts," and that is reflected in the sheer number of hydrocodone and acetaminophen products on the market. Hydrocodone is perhaps the most prescribed narcotic painkiller in the country, and combined with the over the counter medicine acetaminophen (Tylenol), it is available in no less than seventeen different strengths, which means there ought to be one out there to match with whatever size pain you're up against. Eventually someone got the idea to combine hydrocodone with another over the counter medicine, ibuprofen (Advil, Motrin), and in 1997 Vicoprofen was born. Reprexain is simply the same hydrocodone/ibuprofen combination found in Vicoprofen, with the difference being in the strength of hydrocodone per tablet.

The Scam

You could make an argument that Vicoprofen, available in only one strength, 7.5 milligrams of hydrocodone and 200 milligrams of ibuprofen, limits a prescriber's choices when trying to match the right strength of medicine to the level of pain being treated, and that Reprexain, which comes in 2.5/200, 5/200, and 10/200 varieties, provides some needed options when picking a pain med. The thing is, concern for these types of problems only seems to come up when there is money to be made. Vicoprofen is now old enough that is available in a generic form that will cost you around $50 for a hundred tablets. Hawthorn Pharmaceuticals, makers of Reprexain, holds a patent for the *strengths* of the medicines in its tablets, not for the medicines themselves. This means there aren't and won't be any generics for the 2.5, 5, or 10/200 strengths until those patents expire.

The bottom line? If you get a prescription for Reprexain 2.5/200, which is a weaker version of the generic Vicoprofen tablets, you'll pay around $80. You read that right, you will literally be paying more for less.

What To Do

If your prescriber hands you a prescription for Reprexain, ask her if she thinks Vicoprofen would work for you, or better yet, ask if she thinks using Tylenol instead of ibuprofen would make that much of a difference in your treatment. If not, you'd be able to use one of the various hydrocodone/acetaminophen combinations I mentioned earlier and save around 60% compared to what you'd pay for a Reprexain prescription.

And even if your prescriber thinks ibuprofen is your way to go, there's no reason you have to get it in a prescription product. You can go to the pain reliever section of any drugstore and pick up 200 mg ibuprofen tablets for a few dollars. There are very few people for whom a Reprexain prescription justifies the price. Talk to your prescriber about your options. Chances are your wallet will thank you.

Chapter 38: Rezira

The Med

I've heard it said that coughs and colds are to healthcare professionals what divorce is to those who work with the law -a steady source of income and assurance of a continued livelihood. Cough...cough...I have a bit of a respiratory infection going on as I write this, and I can totally understand...cough cough. While I know that...cough cough...this bug will run its course, that it can be expected to last up to 2 weeks if left untreated or 14 days if I take some medicine, boy I would love to have some relief, and boy would I be willing to pay some money for a product that could give it to me. Hawthorn Pharmaceuticals Inc. hopes to get a piece of my money with Rezira, a combination of hydrocodone, used here as a cough suppressant, and pseudoephedrine, a nasal decongestant. As miserable as I feel right now, they won't...cough cough...get it.

The Scam

Because, as many of you probably noticed already, there is nothing new about hydrocodone or pseudoephedrine. The former is among the most commonly prescribed medicines in the country, most popularly as the pain reliever Vicodin, which combines hydrocodone with the over the counter acetaminophen

(Tylenol) we all know and love, while pseudoephedrine has been around for generations as Sudafed. You should be able to get a box along with a prescription for Vicodin and spend less than $20. Show up at the pharmacy counter with an order for Rezira though, and you'll walk away around $60 poorer.

But here's the kicker. The acetaminophen that's in Vicodin but not Rezira would work as an additional pain reliever, as well as against a fever. Rezira has nothing in it to help with fever, so with Rezira, you're actually paying more for less. Cough cough...that wasn't the sound of my cold, that was people all over the country with prescriptions coughing up dollars they don't have to. The burning up however, whether because they realized how much they've spent unnecessarily or due to their untreated fever, will be totally silent though.

What To Do

If you get a prescription for Rezira, ask your doctor for original formula Vicodin instead. (The words "original formula" are important here.You'll see why later.) If your doctor seems confused as to why you're asking for a pain reliever, ask him to look up the active ingredients of both products. Then if you have a fever and want to have a little fun, ask him why he wasn't going to do anything about your elevated temperature. After he stutters and stammers around for an explanation, take your Vicodin prescription to the pharmacy and ask the clerk for a box of original

Sudafed. In 2006 the federal government mandated that all pseudoephedrine be moved behind the counter and signed for, but it is still the same nasal decongestant that has been used for decades (do NOT buy the "Sudafed PE" you find in the cough and cold section that doesn't require a signature. This was brought to market in response to the increased pseudoephedrine regulations, and I have yet to have a customer tell me it works). On your way home you can buy some chicken soup or other cold remedies with the money you've saved. It should help your cold go away in about 2 weeks, or maybe 14 days.

Chapter 39: Rybix ODT

The Med

We'll stay in the world of pain for this one, because in a world where everybody hurts, there is no shortage of ways for a drug company to take advantage to enrich itself. Rybix is a form of the popular painkiller tramadol, known to many all over the country as the brand name Ultram. More than 18 million prescriptions a year are written for Ultram, which is now available as an inexpensive generic. If you've gotten this far in the book though, you're probably aware that effective, popular, and cheap is not a combination the pharmaceutical industry will tolerate if they can do anything about it.

The Scam

Rybix ODT is the same drug that is in the Ultram so many prescribers and patients have become familiar with. It is the same strength; it has the same side effects, and works on the same pain receptors in the body. The only difference is that Rybix ODT is a tablet that dissolves on the tongue (the ODT stands for "orally disintegrating tablet"), as opposed to being swallowed the traditional way. You might think this delivery system sounds like a great idea, as people in pain generally want it to go away as soon as possible, and having the tablet melt in your mouth would save some time. Tramadol doesn't fully start to kick in though, until it is metabolized into a stronger form by the liver, and dissolving tramadol under the tongue doesn't get it metabolized and out of the liver much faster than just swallowing it. Indeed, Shionogi Inc., the maker of Rybix ODT, doesn't claim that it works any faster. The pitch on its advertising materials says only:

> Rybix ODT is the first and only tramadol available in an orally disintegrating tablet. You simply place the tablet on your tongue and wait for it to dissolve—no water needed. That means you can get the pain relief you need wherever you are—even when there's no water handy.

Which would be great I suppose, if pain were to strike you somewhere in the middle of the Sahara desert. Most of us though, have ready access to water, and most of us also value our money. A hundred tablets of Rybix ODT will cost you or your insurance company over $275. A hundred regular tramadol tablets costs less than $20, plus whatever you'd have to pay for a glass of water.

What To Do

If you're Donald Trump, or another person likely to see your prescription medication as a status symbol, of if you're hurting and lost in the middle of an extremely arid part of the planet, then Rybix ODT may be the med for you. Otherwise there's no reason to use Rybix ODT. Like I wrote earlier, it is the same med in the same strength as the tramadol tablets that are on the fast-mover rack of every pharmacy in the country. If your prescriber hands you a prescription for Rybix, asking for tramadol instead just might save you enough to cover the cost of your office visit.

Chapter 40: Sarafem

The Med

PMS is the Rodney Dangerfield of the medical world. Mocked and made fun of, used as both a punchline and a tool of the misogynistic, so often not taken seriously. I'm sure it's no laughing matter to the women who cope with PMS every month though, or the estimated 3 to 8 percent of women who deal with the sadness, despair, anxiety, sleep disturbances, chronic fatigue, difficulty concentrating and other symptoms of PMS' more severe form, Premenstrual Dysphoric Disorder, or PMDD. Being a woman isn't easy sometimes. And then there's the labor pains and the whole childbirth thing.

If those PMDD symptoms sounded a lot like depression to you though, you would be right. It is theorized that PMDD is a result of altered levels in the body of the chemical serotonin, which is also responsible for cases of depression and related disorders, and eventually a class of antidepressants that increase levels of serotonin, known as SSRIs, began to be used in the treatment of PMDD with good results. Sarafem, a brand name of the SSRI fluoxetine, is the only prescription medicine marketed exclusively as a treatment for PMDD.

The Scam

Sarafem is not the only SSRI used for PMDD though. Nor is it even the only version of fluoxetine on the market. Some of you may already recognize the name fluoxetine as the generic version of Prozac, one of the few prescription medicines to break through the medical world to become, like Valium or Viagra, a cultural icon in itself. Prozac and the other SSRI's used to treat PMDD, sertraline (Zoloft), paroxetine (Paxil), and escitalopram (Lexapro), have been around long enough that they are all available as cheap generics. You should be able to get any of them for less than $10 a month.

Cheap is not a word you would use to describe Sarafem though. Its maker, Warner Chilcott, holds a patent not on the medicine fluoxetine itself, but on the use of fluoxetine in the treatment of PMDD. Which means it can make its own version of fluoxetine, and even though it is the same med and same strength as the inexpensive generic Prozac, they market it as the only approved fluoxetine for PMDD. Because of these legalities, if your prescriber gives you a prescription for Sarafem, I or anyone else manning the pharmacy counter cannot use that $10 fluoxetine without getting the prescription changed. We would have to use Sarafem, and only Sarafem.

And we'd have to charge you around $250 a month.

What To Do

Unless you're worried about someone going through your medicine cabinet, finding a prescription with the word "Prozac" somewhere on the label, and thinking you might be depressed, obsessive compulsive, panicky or bulimic, if your prescriber gives you a prescription for Sarafem, ask them for one for generic fluoxetine instead. It's the same med and the same strength, and will cost you around $240 a month less. With an extra $2880 a year, you could probably afford a new medicine cabinet away from prying eyes, or maybe even a whole new bathroom.

Chapter 41: Solodyn

The Med

Solodyn is a version of the popular antibiotic minocycline, which is used to treat a wide variety of infections. The promiscuous among you might be happy to know it can be used for gonorrhea, syphilis, and chlamydia. To the outdoor enthusiasts, that it can treat Rocky Mountain Spotted Fever. To history buffs, that it counters bubonic plague. Minocycline is one of the most versatile antibiotics on the market, but the makers of Solodyn, Medicis Pharmaceutical, are interested in only one type of patient; people with acne. Preferably people with acne and either very good prescription insurance or whose self esteem issues will lead them to the conclusion that money is no object.

The Scam

Traditional minocycline has been available in 50 and 100 milligram strengths since long before I started behind the pharmacy counter, and isn't terribly expensive. You shouldn't pay more than $30 or so for a month's supply. Solodyn, though, is different. How different? Instead of those 50 or 100 milligrams, with Solodyn you'll be getting 55 or 105 milligrams. That's right, five extra measly milligrams. Or 65, 80, or 115 milligrams if those suit you or your doctor's fancy. And instead of the twice a day traditional minocycline dose, Solodyn is an extended-release tablet, so you take it once a day. All for a price of over $800 a month. Same medicine, $730 extra dollars. That's Solodyn in a nutshell.

But wait, if you look at the Solodyn web site, you'll find an offer for big savings! For those of you without insurance, the Medicis MediSAVE program will lower your out of pocket prescription cost for Solodyn to $50! Which while over $700 off full retail price, is still around $20 more a month than what you'll probably pay for regular minocycline. And if you do have insurance and don't mind sticking your insurance company with a $780 tab, you can pay just $20 a month for your Solodyn, but only for three out of every six months. Those other three months you're on your own. Good luck.

What To Do

There's no reason for Solodyn to exist, other than to cure "more money than brains" disease. Medicis will imply its variety of dosage strengths allow your prescriber to give you a lower total dose, which will lower your chances for side effects. There haven't been any studies that I know of that compare the rate of side effects of 50 mg of minocycline twice a day vs that of 105 mg once a day, but I'll go out on a limb and say that any differences would be incredibly minor. And by incredibly minor I mean nonexistent. And if you do have side effects with minocycline, chances are your doctor can simply switch you to another, inexpensive alternative. There is no shortage of acne treatments available in this country after all.

So if your prescriber hands you a prescription for Solodyn, ask her why she thinks it's worth over $9500 a year, and unless you get a really good answer, ask for a prescription for the regular minocycline instead.

Chapter 42: Sular

The Med

The American hypertension market is huge, with over 68 million people in this country, or almost one in three adults, classified as having high blood pressure. Accompanying that high blood pressure is an increased risk of heart attack, stroke, heart failure and kidney disease. Hypertension is a primary or contributing cause of death for over 300,000 Americans a year and costs the country an estimated $131 billion a year in direct medical expenses. With a market like that, it must have seemed to the drug companies that developing an antihypertensive medicine, any antihypertensive medicine, would be a can't-miss moneymaking opportunity. Indeed, I can remember a time when pretty much any drug to treat high blood pressure that made it to market was a guaranteed blockbuster. Gradually though, the market became saturated, with dozens of different products from many different classes of drugs on the market today for your doctor to choose from. Sular came to the party just a little too late. A member of what's called the calcium channel blockers, this perfectly acceptable med was just never able to carve out a niche for itself in a crowded field. Sular languished on most drugstore shelves for a few years until it was old enough to be made generically, which for most brand name meds signals the end of their product life cycle.

The Scam

However, Shionogi Inc, the makers of Sular, aren't ones to give up so easily. If a product just is never going to sell in the volume required to give you a nice profit in the free marketplace, what's a drug company to do? In Shionogi's case the answer is simple: change the market. When it became clear the old Sular was going to be a commercial dud, it was discontinued, and was replaced with "new" Sular. The old 10, 20, 30, and 40 milligram strengths were discontinued, and 8.5, 17, 25.5, and 34 milligram versions took their place. It was like Shionogi had a monopoly on Sular all over again, as there were no generic versions on the market for these new strengths.

And what were the clinical advantages of these new versions of the old med? None. The financial advantages though, were enormous, as new Sular sells for over $350 a month. The "money saving" generics eventually caught up with the new Sular, and can be had for around $175, which sounds like a deal, until you dig a little deeper.

What To Do

Most of the time, when a person needs a particular drug, and that drug is very expensive, that person has little choice but to dig deep into their pocketbook and cough up the money. Remember though, the blood pressure market is huge, with those dozens of products I mentioned earlier. One of those products is a medicine by the name of Norvasc, which did manage to carve out a huge piece of the blood pressure business for itself. It is what's called a dihydropyridine calcium channel blocker, just like Sular. It is so similar that your body probably can't tell the difference between one and the other. Your wallet can though. Pfizer made enough money off of Norvasc back in the day that they didn't feel the need to play the "new strength" game with it when it went generic, (even though you might remember from the chapter on Caduet they did try the "combination product" trick) which means you can get a month's worth of amlodipine, the generic version of Norvasc, for easily under $10.

If your prescriber tries to give you a prescription for Sular, ask her if there's any reason why you can't use Norvasc instead. If she can give you one that's worth $1980 a year, then by all means stick with the Sular. I have a feeling that an extra couple grand in your pocket just might do wonders for keeping your blood pressure down though.

Chapter 43: Treximet

The Med

Treximet is a combination of two different medicines, sumatriptan and naproxen. Sumatriptan was a breakthrough in the treatment of migraine headaches when it was introduced under the brand name of Imitrex in 1991. It was different, and for many people suffering from debilitating migraines, more effective than any of the options previously available. Imitrex soon became a blockbuster drug and a mainstay in the medicine cabinets of many who battle migraines. Naproxen is one of the most commonly used pain relievers in the country. It's in the medicine cabinets of millions who suffer from pain of all sorts. It is a close relative of the over the counter pain relieving staple ibuprofen, and is available over the counter as well, under the name Aleve.

The Scam

In case you haven't caught on yet, Treximet is nothing more than the addition of an over the counter pain reliever to a prescription medicine for migraine headaches. Naproxen and its cousin ibuprofen are in the over the counter pain relieving section of every drugstore in America, cheap and ready to buy. A bottle of 100 tablets will cost you around eight dollars on drugstore.com for example.

Sumatriptan is also pretty cheap since GlaxoSmithKline's patient for it expired. A prescription for 9 tablets, the most commonly prescribed quantity, will cost you somewhere around $25. So a combination of naproxen and sumatriptan should run you around $33.

Get a prescription for Treximet though, and you'll pay close to $220. Which is enough to give me a headache just thinking about it.

What To Do

Pozen Incorporated, which markets Treximet along with GlaxoSmithKline, says on its website that "Treximet has been shown to provide superior sustained pain relief compared to placebo and to both of the single mechanism of action components." They're probably hoping you don't read that very carefully, because what they're saying is that a combination of sumatriptan and naproxen has been shown to work better than 1) nothing at all 2) treating your migraine with only sumatriptan or 3) only naproxen. What they don't mention and what they hope you don't realize is that Treximet isn't the only way to get a combination of these two drugs. If your prescriber wants to give you a prescription for Treximet, just ask for one for Imitrex instead. Treximet uses 85 milligrams of sumatriptan, while Imitrex comes in 50 and 100mg versions. So if you get a prescription for 100mg you'll actually have something *stronger* than Treximet. Then, head to the over the counter pain relievers and pick up some naproxen or ibuprofen, and end your migraine without emptying your wallet.

Chapter 44: Veramyst

The Med

Ahhhhh......ahhhhhhh....ahhhhhhhhh CHOOOOOOO!! If you're making that sound when the pollen hits the air you are far from alone. There is big money to be made in the sneezes, sniffles, and runny noses of allergy season, as evidenced by the over the counter allergy section full of Benadryl, Claritin, Chlor-Trimeton, Nasalcrom, Zyrtec, Alavert, Tavist, and others found in every drugstore in the country. Behind the pharmacy counter it's the same way, as Veramyst, the brand name of a drug called fluticasone furoate competes in a crowded field of prescription allergy meds meant to keep you sneeze and sniffle free. What is the Veramyst difference? The furoate.

The Scam

Some of you may already be familiar with fluticasone *propionate,* a nasal spray that has been sold under the brand name of Flonase for years. Fluticasone *propionate* has been a blockbuster drug and a godsend to millions of allergy sufferers. So what is the difference between fluticasone *propionate* and the fluticasone *furoate* found in Veramyst? It's a different salt.

Please don't read that and try to put Veramyst on your french fries. I'm not talking about table salt. But just as the white crystals in your salt shaker dissolve into sodium and chloride ions upon contact with water, Flonase will dissolve into fluticasone and propionate ions, and Veramyst into fluticasone and furoate.

What I'm about to say next will sound familiar to those of you who remember the Pexeva/Paxil scam I talked about earlier. The thing is, it's only the fluticasone that relieves your allergy symptoms. Your body doesn't care if something dissolves into fluticasone and furoate or fluticasone and pure gold; it's only interested in the fluticasone ions to stop your allergies.

Pure gold might not be a bad thing to have if you get a Veramyst prescription though, as it will most likely cost you over $120 a month. Flonase, which is now available as a generic and sprays the exact same fluticasone ions into your nose, will run you around $20.

What To Do

You know who agrees with me when I say Veramyst is essentially Flonase in a fancier box? The drug reps who are out there selling Veramyst. It didn't take me very long on the Google to find an internet forum full of comments from drug reps saying what they *really* think about their products. My favorite Veramyst comment from cafepharma.com:

"There is a huge difference, Flonase comes in an amber glass bottle and was a class leader along with mometasone (Nasonex) in efficacy. Veramyst is our leftover Flonase bottles with a plastic shell around it to make sure that when you drop your Flonase bottle it does not shatter. We have that different side chain to (sic) which has no clinical relevance as stated in our own PI...oh and Veramyst will cost you 3 times as much minimum per month as generic Flonase and twice as much as Nasonex."

Cut out the industry jargon and it's pretty clear what this sales rep thinks of the product. I'm betting the doctors she calls on don't get this version.

So evidently pharmaceutical sales reps and I have finally found a point of agreement. If you get a prescription for Veramyst, ask your doctor for Flonase instead. Or hope for some fluticasone that dissolves into solid gold.

Chapter 45: Vicodin

The Med

Vicodin, a combination of the narcotic pain reliever hydrocodone and over the counter acetaminophen, is the most commonly prescribed drug in the country, with over 130 million prescriptions written for it and all its generic forms in 2010 according to WebMd.com. If you've ever had a wisdom tooth pulled, sprained an ankle or broken an arm, or otherwise found yourself in a world of hurt, chances are you've used Vicodin to ease your pain. Just not the Vicodin I'm talking about. Today's Vicodin, according to its manufacturer Abbott labs, has been "improved." Today's Vicodin is easier on your liver, but a lot harder on your pocketbook than it has to be.

The Scam

One of my biggest pet peeves in my years behind the pharmacy counter was when I would see a prescription for the old Vicodin, which contained 500 milligrams of acetaminophen per tablet, with instructions of "Take one to two tablets every four to six hours." There aren't as many hard and fast rules in medicine as you might imagine, that's why they use the term "practicing" after all, but there is a very clear upper limit to the amount of acetaminophen a person should have a day, and it is 4000mg. Any more than that and a person risks damaging the liver, whose job it is to metabolize and eventually get rid of all the acetaminophen we put into our bodies. Do the math and you'll see that a person taking two of the old Vicodin tablets every four hours would end up with 2000mg more than the maximum daily acetaminophen dose. Yet those same set of instructions would roll in day after day, all day long. I solved the problem by starting to type "No more than eight tablets a day" on the label, which once led to an angry phone call from a doctor wanting to know who I thought I was to change his directions. I explained some simple arithmetic to him and waited for his thank you, which came in the form as an unintelligible grunt before he hung up the phone.

Eventually though, concern about excess acetaminophen dosing started to spread, and even the government caught wind of the potential problems, with the FDA asking drug manufacturers to limit the amount of acetaminophen in their products.

Abbott was happy to comply, reducing the amount of acetaminophen in a tablet of Vicodin from 500 to 300 milligrams. Purely out of concern for the condition of the public's livers I'm sure. The fact that this new strength would not have as many generic competitors, and therefore the price of a 30 tablet Vicodin prescription would go from around $12 to over $50 was just a consequence of the research it took to figure out how to put less of something in the same tablet I'm sure.

But wait, because this story gets even better.

The old Vicodin had for many years a competitor that went by the name of Norco. Just like Vicodin, Norco was a combination of hydrocodone and acetaminophen, and was available in many different strengths, all of which though, featured 325mg of acetaminophen.

To put this another way, there was always an option for doctors who wanted to use a lower dose of acetaminophen, and when Abbott made a big deal of lowering the amount in Vicodin, they picked a strength that was just 25mg lower than what was already on the market, and that sold for around $18.

What To Do

If a prescriber wants to hand you a prescription for today's Vicodin, ask for Norco instead. What you'll be getting is 25mg more of acetaminophen per tablet, which a healthy and normally functioning liver won't even notice, and about $30 more in your pocket.

Chapter 46: Vusion Ointment

The Med

They say the bond between parent and child is the strongest a human can form, and something that a childless person can never quite understand. Having no children myself, I suppose I'll never know, but I'm pretty sure that's probably right. Evolution would have to create a pretty damn strong bond to withstand the noisy, smelly, mess making, mess getting into, sleep depriving experience that is parenthood after all. I've worked in a retail setting for close to 25 years, which means I now see babies who could be the babies of the first little tyrants I saw wailing down the toy aisle long ago, and I am convinced. To put up with one of those things you would have to love them. A lot.

I bet the people at Stiefel Laboratories understand that as well. That a few of them are even parents, and that on occasion, they have experienced the unique horror that must come from seeing the child you love so much with its butt on fire. I'm talking about diaper rash, and I'm not trying to minimize the condition. I'm sure it's awful for a little guy or girl to have to go through. I'm also sure that the first reaction of most parents would be something along the lines of "I NEED TO DO SOMETHING!!!!!" That the sight of such suffering, along with a tinge of guilt that would come from thinking maybe they had had something to do with this, *"Did I change the diapers enough? Was I not diligent enough with the baby powder?"* would spur a parent to do anything in their power to make things right again.

That's how most parents would think that is. The parents who work at Stiefel Laboratories evidently thought something along the lines of "We could make some money off of this. A literal buttload of money," which would explain the creation of Vusion ointment.

The Scam

It's not that Vusion is ineffective. It never would have been approved unless there was evidence that it worked. The product's package insert lists three ingredients; miconazole, zinc oxide, and white petrolatum.

Miconazole is an antifungal agent used to treat secondary yeast infections that can take hold during an episode of diaper rash. It's good stuff to use in these situations, and Vusion contains it in a concentration of 0.25%

Thing is, you can buy an over the counter tube of miconazole, eight times as strong, in the athlete's foot aisle. It goes by the name of Micatin.

Zinc Oxide is a skin protectant that also helps to seal

out moisture. Again, a great idea to use when skin is irritated and wet. You'll get it in a concentration of 15% in Vusion. Or you could get some over the counter Desitin and get it in a concentration of 40%.

The audacity to list white petrolatum as an active ingredient is my favorite. White petrolatum is Vaseline.

So, let's recap. Vusion is a prescription product that contains a combination of ingredients in weaker strengths than you can find them over the counter. Now let's do some math:

One tube Micatin, 14grams, $6.49 (all prices from drugstore.com).

One tube Desitin, 120 grams, $4.42.

Vaseline, 75 grams, $3.29.

Which gives us a grand total of $14.20.

So, how much do you suppose a prescription of Vusion goes for, after you go through the process of being examined by a licensed prescriber and given the right to buy something not as strong? Guess. Seriously... before you read any farther, I want you to take a stab at how much you think the good folks at Stiefel laboratories will charge you for watered down over the counter products.

Ready?

$265.99 for a 50 gram tube. I am not making that up.

So by all means, the next time you gasp in horror when you realize your little one's butt is in an awful way, ask your doctor if Vusion is right for you, and if your doctor says yes, find another doctor.

What To Do

As you can see, a do it yourself, more effective version of Vusion can easily be mixed together at home. If you can't find Micatin, another over the counter antifungal such as Lotrimin (clotrimazole) or Lamisil (terbinafine) will do the trick. Whip up a batch and you'll soon discover that defeating diaper rash is probably the easiest of the parenting problems you'll face over the next 20 years or so.

Chapter 47: Xerese

The Med

Here's a true fact that will more than likely scare some of you. You and almost everyone you meet has been exposed to the herpes virus. Don't let that put a crimp in your social life though, because it doesn't have a thing to do with promiscuity. I'm talking about cold sores, which are caused by the herpes simplex virus type 1, and not the genital herpes which is caused by the type 2 virus and usually acquired in ways that are more fun. In about a third of us, that initial exposure to the type 1 virus will lead to recurrent, periodic outbreaks of those tingly, painful and unsightly cold sores. I always thought it a bit ironic that infection with type 1 herpes can decrease your likelihood of being exposed to type 2. Fortunately for most of us, cold sores are just an annoyance, and there are treatment options available. Xerese is a prescription cream that combines an antiviral drug, acyclovir, with the well known and commonly used anti-inflammatory med hydrocortisone.

The Scam

Xerese was far from a breakthrough when it hit the market in May of 2011. Acyclovir had been around for years in both topical and tablet form, and all Xerese did was add the same hydrocortisone found in the first aid aisle of every drugstore in the country. How much could an underwhelming innovation like that be worth really?

Do you want to take a guess before I tell you?

Right around $350 dollars for a five gram tube. In case you're not up your metric system, imagine the length of the first two joints of your pinky finger, with half the circumference, and you'll have an idea how big a five gram tube is.

If you go to the website for Xerese though, you'll see a "pay no more than $15" coupon, and if you hate your insurance company and want to give them a reason to jack up your premiums at renewal time, you can certainly take advantage of this offer. Read the fine print very carefully though, because there's a good chance that when you use the "pay no more than $15" card you'll be paying more than $15. If you're uninsured you'll definitely be paying far more than $15.

Some of you may be thinking you can just use the acyclovir cream that's been around forever and buy some hydrocortisone on your own. And you can. Except that the company that makes Xerese, Valeant Dermatology, also bought the rights to make the only acyclovir cream on the market, Zovirax. A tube of Zovirax will run you around $350 as well.

So what's a cold sore sufferer to do? Buy something

more effective, for less money. That's what.

<u>What To Do</u>

The thing is, treating a cold sore topically is not your only option. There are also oral prescription medicines that can be used for cold sores.

And they work better.

Here's the deal. According to the trade publication *Pharmacist's Letter,* treatment with regular acyclovir cream will make a cold sore go away about a day sooner than it otherwise would. Add a little hydrocortisone the way Xerese does and you can make that a day and a half. If you can remember to constantly apply the stuff five times a day that is.

A prescription for oral acyclovir though, will get that thing off your face up to two days quicker. And cost you around $12.

Did you get that? More effective, and $338 less. And if you'd rather not have to worry about taking something five times a day, you can use a related drug, valacyclovir, which is taken just two times and will cost you around $25.

So if your doctor tries to give you a prescription for Xerese, just ask for acyclovir or valacyclovir instead. You'll get better results and have more in your wallet.

And you'll look smarter than a doctor, once that cold sore clears up.

Chapter 48: Zipsor

The Med

Bruises, bumps, burns, and sprains. Those are just some of life's painful surprises a person can expect to deal with at some point. Zipsor promises relief for those and other acute painful situations using "The efficacy of diclofenac and the efficiency of ProSorb® drug delivery in a single solution," according to its website. Sounds impressive to be sure, but what exactly does that mean?

Diclofenac is a pain reliever and inflammatory that's been busting the pain for years under the brand name of Voltaren. The Zipsor difference is that it's a liquid filled capsule, instead of a traditional tablet. It's the same medicine and the same strength (the lowest available) as you get with the generic versions of Voltaren. It's just in a liquid filled capsule.

The Scam

So does that matter? The makers of Zipsor, Depomed Inc., never really tell you. The fact that Zipsor is "the first prescription nonsteroidal anti-inflammatory drug with ProSorb® dispersion technology" certainly *sounds* impressive, but any proof ProSorb® makes the slightest bit of difference in how diclofenac actually works is conspicuously absent. The only study cited in the official prescribing information for Zipsor compares it to a placebo, so we know that Zipsor handily beats using nothing for pain relief, but as far as how it compares with a regular diclofenac tablet? Not a word.

Of course that doesn't mean Zipsor isn't a little quicker at getting into your bloodstream, which is what the people at Depomed would want you to believe. Ask yourself a question though, if there was any evidence of this, anything at all a PR or advertising firm could grab a hold of and put up on that web page or any of the other advertising for Zipsor to show it actually worked better or faster...

...don't you think they would have done it? Either there's no evidence of any Zipsor advantage or Depomed has hired the worst advertising agency in the world. I'll let you decide which is more likely.

Now ask yourself another question, is the mere implication, a hopeful suggestion, though not an outright claim, that a med might be somewhat better than an alternative worth paying $80 for? Because that's the approximate difference between the price of 30 Zipsor capsules compared to 30 diclofenac tablets.

The people at Depomed hope your answer is yes. Your wallet, however, is seriously rooting against that.

What To Do

Unless you feel like starting your own economic stimulus program by pumping some excess dollars into the economy, if your prescriber brings up the subject of Zipsor, change the conversation to regular diclofenac instead. You may help to create a recession for Depomed, but you'll be laying the groundwork for a bright economic future for a person that matters; you.

Chapter 49: Ziana

The Med

If you've been reading the whole book to this point, one thing you've undoubtedly learned is that there is no shortage of prescription products that are slightly manipulated versions of long available and inexpensive acne treatments that are highly marked up. I started this book with Acanya, and now with Ziana, we can say the pimple rip offs literally go from A to Z. Ziana is yet another combination of two previously available acne treatments, this time the antibiotic clindamycin (found here in a slightly different strength, 1.2%, as opposed to the widely used 1% version) and tretinoin, which has been sold for years under the brand name Retin-A.

The Scam

Other than the slight modification of the clindamycin strength, which was done with no clinical evidence that 1.2% works any better than the 1% that has always been used, there is nothing new or unique about Ziana. It is simply a combination of two medicines in one cream. Ziana makes no claim to work any better or have fewer side effects than any of the options to treat acne that were on the market before it. There is a section on the product's website called "Why Ziana Gel?" and the best they can come up with is that it "offers these demonstrated acne fighters in one easy-to-use gel," and that it's not sticky. I suppose the fact that Ziana is not sticky is a good thing, but I have to be honest, I've never taken stickiness into consideration when making medical decisions.

Of course to buy two separate prescriptions of the topical clindamycin and tretinoin can be kinda pricey. You can expect to pay around $90 to treat your acne this way, which seems high, until you price a 60 gram tube of Ziana.

Ziana will run you or your insurance company over $400. Taking two non-sticky products and combining them into one non-sticky product is a very expensive proposition evidently. There is a "money saving" offer on Ziana's website that will allow you to shift everything but $20 to your insurance company, but boy that's going to make them mad. Mad enough to remember you when it's time to set your premium for the next year I bet.

And if you're uninsured, that "savings card" will knock the price of a tube of Ziana down to $50, but only for your first three tubes. After that you're on your own.

What to do

Skip the Ziana, and go with one of the other non-sticky alternatives. If separate prescriptions of clindamycin and tretinoin are still a little pricey for your budget, ask your doctor about using another antibiotic in place of the clindamycin. A tube of topical erythromycin, for instance, will run you around $15, which means you can use that with the tretinoin and still end up paying less than a tube of Ziana with the "savings card."

Bottom line: treating acne doesn't have to be expensive, despite the drug company's efforts to make you think so. If your doctor is draining your pocketbook while zapping your pimples, show them this book.

Chapter 50: For The Sake Of Completeness, An Over The Counter Rip Off. ZzzQuil.

The Med

Remember NyQuil? "The nighttime, sniffling, sneezing, coughing, aching, stuffy head, fever so you can rest medicine," the old slogan went, and that's how millions of people used it over the years, not so much to get relief from their cough and cold symptoms, but just to knock themselves out so they could get some sleep while they felt miserable. ZzzQuil aims to take advantage of the coma-inducing reputation of NyQuil, and you'll see it packaged in the same colors and font of its famous cold medicine cousin, no doubt to make you think of the good night's sleep you got the last time you used NyQuil. ZzzQuil strips out the nasal decongestant, cough suppressant, and pain reliever and leaves just an antihistamine, which was used to treat sneezing and runny noses in NyQuil, but which also has a side effect of making a person drowsy. Change the label a bit, and now you have a sleep aid

The Scam

Except ZzzQuil uses a *different* antihistamine than the one used in NyQuil. Diphenhydramine is the med you'll find in ZzzQuil, which is a relative of the doxylamine used in NyQuil. While it's kinda odd that Proctor and Gamble, maker of both ZzzQuil and NyQuil, would choose a different med to make you sleepy, the thing is

doxylamine is stronger than diphenhydramine.

I am not making this up. For whatever reason, P&G decided to take advantage of the sleep-inducing reputation of one of its products by coming out with something that is officially labeled for sleep, but doesn't work as well.

And that drug was also already available in several forms. The popular over the counter sleep aid Nytol uses diphenhydramine. As does almost every other over the counter sleep aid in the drugstore with the exception of original Unisom. Got that? If you want the sleep inducing properties of NyQuil without the other cold meds and pain reliever, you have to buy not ZzzQuil, but a different brand made by an entirely different company.

And just to make things more complicated, diphenhydramine is also sold as an allergy medicine. It's the ingredient in the original Benadryl allergy.

It's complicated I know, and all you want to do is get some sleep. I'll make it easy for you.

<u>What To Do</u>

Forget the Zzzquil. As a matter of fact, forget everything you know about over the counter sleep aids except for the rest of this paragraph. Diphenhydramine will make you drowsy, and it wears off quicker. If you're worried about still being groggy in the morning, use diphenhydramine to sleep. But not for more than a few days, as the effects will wear off.

Doxylamine will make you more drowsy, but there is a chance you might still be groggy in the morning. Also, the effects of doxylamine don't diminish over time the way diphenhydramine does. If you want something stronger, or find yourself needing a sleep aid often, doxylamine may be a better choice.

And Zzzquil has no reason to exist. Just like every other drug you've just read about.

It's a jungle out there in the healthcare world, and there is no shortage of ways for your doctor to hand you a slip of paper that separates you from a good chunk of your money for no good reason. Just remember, your interest as a patient is to get better, while the interest of the drug companies is to vacuum up every last dollar they possibly can. Sometimes those interests will coincide, but many times they will not.

Be careful out there. And never be afraid to do a little research.

Good luck.

Made in the USA
Lexington, KY
06 September 2013